Walk For Your Life! presents a refreshing ov~~erview~~ our physical environment impacts our quality ~~... cap~~tured how the ability to walk where we live, ~~...~~ sense of freedom and the ability to appreciate, interact, and be a part of the world around us. Through an experiential lens, walkable mixed-use environments are contrasted with auto dependent sprawling environments. Questions are raised as to the individual and societal benefits of creating and maintaini~~ng~~ ~~...~~re de~~stinations can be~~ ccessed safely and pleasantly on foot. The design of ou~~r~~ ~~co~~mmunities is a direct reflection of our culture and our values. Our desire for space and for automobility is clearly outpacing our concern for the health of the environment and even for our own physical well-being. Understanding how today's and tomorrow's transportation and land use decisions will shape the physical environment of the future is a critical first step towards achieving sustainability through healthy community design."

> *Dr. Lawrence D. Frank*
> *Bombardier Chair in Sustainable Transportation*
> *School of Community and Regional Planning*
> *University of British Columbia*

Marie Demers makes a powerful case against many of the decisions taken over more than half a century by elected officials, urban planners, transportation experts, architects, engineers and builders who focused almost exclusively on convenience and efficiency in designing the built environment in which we live. One of the unintended consequences of their view of a modern city is that it makes the simplest of activities, i.e. walking, dangerous or almost impossible. She reviews compelling evidence indicating that the decline in walking and the increase in passive and sedentary leisure activities translate into a growing prevalence of overweight and obesity with ensuing epidemics of diabetes, heart disease and other ailments. In a provocative series of arguments, she advocates the reconfiguration of our environment and novel public transport priorities to restore a friendly and safe walking environment. Millions of people do not habitually walk because it is perceived as unsafe as suggested by the daily statistics on pedestrian injuries and fatalities. The same is true for children. This is a shameful situation that the present generation of public and business leaders should strive to correct. For them, *Walk for Your Life!* by Dr Marie Demers would be an excellent place to start. They would find in this thought-provoking book information and inspiration.

Dr. Claude Bouchard, Executive Director
Pennington Biomedical Research Center
Baton Rouge, Louisiana

Marie Demers has written us a prescription for our health and well-being, and for the health of our ailing communities: we need to walk more, and to do this we need to make our communities more walkable. This is the obvious and essential solution to many of our problems.

If we make our communities safe, easy and convenient places in which to walk—for people of all ages and abilities—we will have transformed them into great places in which we all can live. Dr. Demers has given us a wake-up call and provided a roadmap to show us the way.

As a planner, as an advocate for walking and bicycling, and most of all, as a grandfather, I thank her. Now, let's get to work!

Bill Wilkinson, AICP, Executive Director
National Center for Bicycling & Walking

WALK FOR YOUR LIFE!

Restoring Neighborhood Walkways
to Enhance Community Life, Improve Street Safety
and Reduce Obesity

Marie Demers, Ph.D.

VITAL HEALTH PUBLISHING

Walk for Your Life!

Published in 2006 by Vital Health Publishing, Ridgefield, CT
Copyright © Marie Demers, 2006

Cover design: On the Dot Designs
Interior book design: Deborah Rust Design
Interior photographs by permission of Guy Langlois, except as noted.
Cover photographs: top left by permission of Portland Oregon Visitors Association;
bottom left and top right, acquired from Project for Public Spaces; bottom right, acquired
from Superstock.

Published by: Vital Health Publishing
PO Box 152
Ridgefield, CT 06877
Orders: 877-VIT-BOOKS
Web site: www.vitalhealthbooks.com
E-mail: info@vitalhealthbooks.com

Disclaimer
Serious diseases should always be treated under medical supervision.
Never delay in seeking medical advice if you have any persisting medical
or psychological condition. The material in this book is for educational
purposes only and is not intended for use in diagnosing or treating
any individual.

Printed in the United States of America

ISBN-10: 1-890612-49-9
ISBN-13: 978-1-890612-49-8
Library of Congress Control Number: 2005931280

g green press INITIATIVE Vital Health Publishing is committed to the goals of the Green Press Initiative and to preserving Endangered
Forests and conserving natural resources. This book is printed on 30% postconsumer recycled paper.

To my brother Paul

CONTENTS

Foreword

This is a book about walking, but it is really about more than walking. It is about what we want our future to be. Will we leave our children a world where obesity and poor health are the norm, or will we do what it takes to create an environment that supports health and wellness? Believe it or not, it all starts with walking.

The health of our population is getting worse each year, with obesity rates up and fitness levels down. In many countries, the majority of adults are already overweight or obese, and children are not far behind. If we don't do something now, we may be headed for a future in which almost everyone is obese and diseases such as diabetes, heart disease, and cancer are rampant.

How did we get here? We can't blame our poor health solely on individual behavior. We have inadvertently created an environment that promotes obesity by discouraging physical activity and encouraging overeating. It is becoming clear, for example, that the way we build many of our communities and the way we design buildings discourages physical activity. We build communities that discourage walking and buildings that discourage stair use, for example. We have "engineered" physical activity out of our lives. We no longer have to be physically active to get through the day. It is almost impossible to maintain a healthy weight with such a low level of physical activity. Our ancestors were not lean because they engaged in a lot of voluntary physical activity, they were lean because they had to be physically active to get food and shelter and for transportation. Solving our obesity problem can't be done unless we can focus both on helping people make better choices about diet and physical activity, and on modifying the environment in which we live to support and sustain these healthier behaviors.

It is easy to be pessimistic about the future, but I remain optimistic that we must and we will do whatever it takes to reverse the epidemic of obesity. I am convinced that we cannot win a war on obesity unless we can increase the physical activity level of the population. Unfortunately, too much of our efforts to address obesity are based on food strategies. Human biology works best when we are physically active, and so many people get so little physical activity that it is impossible to eat sufficiently little food to keep from gaining weight.

What will it take to start turning things around? I believe we can do it with small changes. Individuals can start making some changes to eat a little healthier and to be a little more physically active. At the same time we can make small changes to our environment, making it easier to be physically active and to eat healthier. I have helped start a national weight-gain prevention program, America on the Move (www.americaonthemove.org), to help people make these small changes.

Walk for Your Life is a great resource to show us how to start addressing the obesity epidemic—for individuals and for our society. The good news is that it doesn't take all that much of an increase in physical activity to get us back to the level where we can balance our food intake and our physical activity. Many of you may think you have so far to go in achieving a healthy lifestyle, but start with small changes. Start with putting one foot in the front of the other, and walk.

— *James O. Hill*

Prologue

I s there a simpler or more natural activity than walking? It always seems to be a spectacular event when a child takes its first steps. We celebrate the child's great achievement and cannot wait to tell others about it; its importance even outclasses that of the child's first words. We can all read the pride in the eyes of a child when he or she walks unaided for the first time, taking the first steps toward autonomy and independence.

Years later, as we become more sedentary, we forget the role of walking in our lives. Most of our activities—work, leisure, and transportation—require us to sit for long periods. Meanwhile, our environment has made it more and more difficult for us to go anywhere on foot, and modern amenities encourage us to save our energy. We do not always realize the adverse effects of this induced inactivity. But there is now a lot of evidence that being physically inactive is harmful. Physical activity is crucially important for our health, even if our only activity is walking.

Fortunately, there are small signs of resistance to this state of passivity. They're not obvious yet, and they may not even be conscious, but after many years of observation, I have no doubt about their existence.

The revival of pilgrimages, the vacations spent strolling through the compact old towns of New England, the trips to Disney World, and even the present craze for miniature Christmas villages all contribute to the effort to restore the walkable environment—even if only in the imagination—that most of us have been deprived of during the last decades. It is not an attempt to turn back the clock, but rather to regain an environment built on a human scale. It has nothing to do with being forced to walk, or with replacing other modes of travel with walking; rather, it is about making it easy to walk in our immediate environment, and restoring walking as an efficient and enjoyable mode of transportation.

This book attempts to answer three questions:

- Why did we stop walking?
- What are the consequences of walking less?
- Where do we go from here?

These pages shows how our sedentary lifestyle is slowly killing us, and what we can do about it.

Part 1

An Environment Hostile to Walking

1
Watching Your Step

A pedestrian is a man in danger of his life;
a walker is a man in possession of his soul.
—David McCord

I remember precisely when the idea of this book first came to my mind, and where I was at that specific moment. It was five years ago, on my way to work in the morning. By choice, I had been taking the bus the three-mile distance from my home to my office every working day. It was more convenient for me than driving, especially in winter when snow fell during the night and there was not enough time to shovel the driveway before going to work the following day. At the bus stop, I usually met a bunch of people who, like me, worked in different departments of the government. We did not know much about each other, but we enjoyed talking while waiting for the bus and commuting together, and I really appreciated the moments we shared.

Since I got my first car late in life compared to other people, I was used to walking and biking a lot, not only for leisure or sport, but also for transportation, in my own country as well as in many places around the world. It was part of my philosophy of life, and my way to keep in shape—despite the fact that I was living in Canada, a cold and rainy country.

I guess I owe this inclination to my father, who was a great walker. His life spanned most of the twentieth century and part of the nineteenth, and he reached almost one hundred years of age, walking every day until his death. He went out many times a day for a walk in our small town, or hiked for hours in the woods surrounding it. I often went with him, and these memories are precious to me. He had already covered three quarters of a century when I was born, and I learned a lot from this unusual but rewarding experience. He was one of the first here to get a car in 1908: the famous Ford Model T. He loved inventions and new technologies. But he always remained an active walker. If he had not, he would not have stayed in such great shape for so long, and I would probably not be here telling about it. Walking around the place kept him in physical condition and in touch with the local community. He enjoyed talking with people passing by, and he never experienced a loss of autonomy.

I moved to this neighborhood to be close to everything so I would rarely have to use my car. It never occurred to me to drive if I didn't have to—until one day when I realized I did not feel safe any longer while crossing the street on foot.

On that day, trying to get from the bus stop to my office, I suddenly began to feel like a hunted animal, like a deer during hunting season. As I crossed a two-lane street, I had the sense the cars coming toward me had me in their sights. I even imagined that the drivers accelerated the moment they spotted me. I arrived at work out of breath, feeling I had survived a battle against the traffic. But it was an uneven struggle: me, the pedestrian, fighting for my life; and the drivers, rushing to save time without compromising the integrity of their cars.

This situation happened again and again, almost every time I tried to cross the street, wherever it was, and not only at rush hour when drivers were in a hurry. I risked my life many times a day crossing the street, although I walk pretty fast. "Run for your life" has become the daily leitmotiv of pedestrians. Many are killed or injured, but all suffer from this permanent struggle for survival.

I wondered when things had changed. I was born during the fifties, and I remembered that once it was normal and safe to walk and play in the streets. For me and my friends, the streets and sidewalks were part of our playground. We used them for jump-rope and baseball in summer and hockey in winter. The first sign of spring was when my father began to cut into pieces the thick layer of ice on the sidewalk, so we soon could use our tricycles. I even remember going downhill in summer on a tricycle with no brakes, with no fear of getting hurt by a car. Many of us also remember the tricks we played on adult pedestrians on the sidewalks. There were not so many cars threatening us then. And we spent so much time playing outside that our parents had to call us many times before we finally agreed to come

We may think these signs are designed to protect pedestrians, but in fact they indicate how much our habitat is shrinking.

in for lunch or dinner. We were always in a hurry to go back outside, to continue our exploration of the world around us. Going by myself to buy a Popsicle at the little convenience store two houses away from mine was part of my summer routine, and of my pride as well, since it gave me a feeling of independence. Most of us walked to school, whatever the distance, and there was no traffic around the school building, because parents did not drive their children there.

A few years later, during the sixties, the sidewalks disappeared from the neighborhoods, and the streets got larger. It also became more difficult to cross the streets at the corner, because new intersections were built with a curb radius that made higher speed possible for motor vehicles, but increased the distance between two corners for pedestrians. In fact, in many places, there were no corners left. Now, walking in the street does not feel safe any more, and crossing the street has become a risky enterprise. Streets are dangerous places to stand, especially at rush hour, because of the speeding cars—but they are still dangerous when the traffic is gone, because they are completely deserted. Children are rarely seen playing in the street, and adults seldom walk there either. The dominance of the car is also cynically illustrated by the invasion of some beaches by Jeeps and other motor vehicles, reminding pedestrians that their habitat is shrinking well beyond streets and roads.

How could such a simple and healthy human activity as walking have become so dangerous and unwelcome in just a few decades? As the idea for this book became clearer, I realized that our external world has been arranged in such a way as to make the lives of pedestrians miserable. It is not that the old days were better; it is not that walking should replace driving. Rather, each mode of transportation should find its own place and harmoniously coexist with the other modes. The more people walk to reach destinations close by, for example, the less traffic congestion in the area, as we will see later. Moreover, the more people walk, the safer walking becomes.

Day after day, I faced the same situation. Although fortunately I was not injured in the struggle of cars versus pedestrians, I finally had to concede defeat. Overwhelmed with a feeling of helplessness, I joined the majority of people commuting to work in their cars.

From there, a kind of chain reaction occurred. Instead of biking less than a mile to the open market during the summer months, as I used to do, I found myself taking the car. All the distances I had covered with my bike or on foot began to seem much longer.

I also felt as if I had no time to walk places; I was in a hurry most of the time. Using my car for commuting and for every small trip changed my perception of distance, time, and safety as well. And it changed how I ran errands: two miles in one direction to get my favorite lasagna, five miles in another direction to buy a special cheese I had heard about, and ten more miles to a supermarket to stock up on bathroom necessities. What a strange paradox—all this frenetic activity made me more lazy. And I still did not clearly understand where those five extra pounds came from or why it was so difficult to get rid of them, although I had modified my food habits and reduced my caloric intake.

The only relief from the humiliation and moral conflict I felt as I adopted these new behaviors was writing this book, to explore the problem more deeply and to alert other people to the wrong choices we are all making and the consequences they have in our life.

2
A Walkable Haven

All truly great thoughts are conceived by walking.
—*Friedrich Nietzsche*

At least, I thought, I still had enough presence of mind and good fortune to buy a house in an area built on a human scale, on a quiet street, but only a five-minute walk from almost everything: the grocery store, the laundry, the elementary and high schools, the public tennis court and swimming pool, the church, the hospital, the garage, the florist, the hardware, the bakery, the fish market, the bank, the barber shop, the dentist, the bus stop, dozens of restaurants—good ones!—and a huge shopping center, one of the biggest in Canada.

It was a fully equipped neighborhood where anyone could walk just a few minutes to get fresh bread and croissants every morning, as well as magazines and newspapers from around the world. And the university was twenty minutes away on foot. Added to the proximity of these services, the beach was within fifteen minutes by bike. I had deliberately placed myself in a situation where it would be convenient—and safe—to walk, and where most of the places I needed to go were reachable on foot. Finding a job at a walking distance would be a very easy task, since there was a tremendous variety of workplaces around.

Nowadays, however, the situation is dramatically different for a majority of people.

She has it all, you are probably saying. But anyone could have bought a house here. Mine is neither new nor very expensive, a solid brick house on a 7,000-square-foot lot, surrounded by mature trees offering a lot of privacy, and overlooking an English garden in the back yard (where I attempt to "play God" on one of the days of creation, planting hundreds of my favorite perennial flowers and lots of shrubs). The house is in an old suburb of the first generation, the beginning of the 1950s, when services and workplaces were still part of the neighborhood, where streets connected with each other, making it possible to choose between many routes to get to a destination. There are still sidewalks here, and the neighborhood is populated by familiar individuals. It is a multipurpose neighborhood in which I am exposed to a variety of people: families with young children or teenagers, retired couples, university students, and single persons. Joining them during the day are those who work in one of the local office buildings or stores, or in the hospital close by, so the area is never deserted. It is simply a suburb without the usual sprawl characteristics. And I know how good it feels to call the garage for an appointment and be recognized by my voice, even before saying my name, as "the lady with the black car." Leaving the car there and walking back home five minutes away while they repair it is very convenient. Going to the grocery store and encountering people who live in the same area and wish me a happy New Year is also a pleasant experience. This familiar neighborhood makes me feel part of the community, as well as safe and secure. It makes my life less complicated and gives me more free time for leisure.

There is no garage adjacent to the house, but I do not really need it. Nevertheless, three cars can easily fit in the narrow driveway. My previous house had a garage, but I almost never parked in it, despite the long, snowy winter and the frequent icy rain. Even in below-zero weather, the car stayed outside. Most people who have garages never use them for their cars. What good is it anyway to park inside the garage during a snowstorm, when there is a distance of twenty-five feet between it and the street? A lot of snow to shovel! And if the weather is nice, there is no need for a shelter. It just seems to be a huge storage room for almost anything. After a few years in the garage, all that stuff is good for is a garage sale.

I should confess there is a shadow in this idyllic picture. Just a few miles from here, the reality of sprawl hits me too, at the end of a short urban highway. There was nothing at all there ten years ago, only green fields and a park for outdoor activities such as fishing, swimming, and cycling. I used to bike there, but not any more. Now the area is filled with supersized stores, fast-food restaurants, and monstrous movie theaters, each uglier than the next, all one-story buildings surrounded by huge parking lots, where you cannot even think about going on foot; it is impossible to reach this place other than by car. Once there, it is also dangerous to walk from one store to the next, because there are too many cars around. There were already so many big shopping centers in the area that this new development did not make sense at all. Nevertheless, the parking lots are always full. It is there, so people come—probably because we like to think we save money when buying thirty double-sized rolls of toilet paper at a time. We may save money, in the short run at least, buying all that stuff imported mostly from developing countries, and sold by underpaid employees, but we lose time and energy going there. I always wonder who is making money when the ads tell me I am saving a few pennies.

Going to this area is an awful excursion and a stressful experience, so everyone rushes back home, retreating to the intimacy of the living room, away from fellow citizens. All over the place, these big-box store developments are replacing the shopping centers where people could still walk from store to store, so the trend increasingly restricts walking opportunities. These commercial developments also make the urban landscape the same everywhere, since they are indistinguishable one from another, displaying the same stores and the same ugly architecture. Now, it is even impossible to know what city you are in from such a viewpoint. According to Marshall

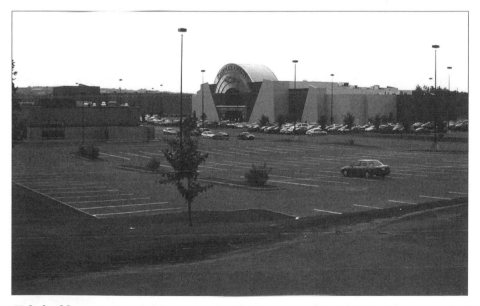

Ugly buildings surrounded by a sea of asphalt are now flourishing in the most recent suburbs—places you cannot walk to, with huge parking lots that are empty most of the time.

McLuhan, whose monumental work on understanding the effects of modern technology is still up to date, "The car gave the American the opportunity, not to travel and experience adventure, but to make himself more and more common."[1]

What you see in this area is a mess spread out over about a two-mile-long strip. I close my eyes and like to imagine instead a nice boulevard with wide sidewalks where a lot of pedestrians are walking and talking to each other, where the traffic is slower; all along the way are higher-density residential developments like townhouses and individual houses on smaller lots, and an activity center, with nice shops offering you special products you cannot find everywhere. So you walk along this boulevard instead of driving; you stop and sit on a bench when you feel tired. You meet some people you know, get the latest news, and go back home relaxed and in better shape, because you did not have to fight for a parking space, and you had an enjoyable walk outside. The store will deliver what you have bought, so you do not even have to carry anything on your way back home. How nice it could be—if we had the choice!

I can already hear the advocates of the American dream, pretending that what most people want is a spacious house on a large lot in a quiet neighborhood away from the hassles of the city, and that sprawl is the only possible answer to their wishes. However, the truth is somewhat different—not only about the dream, but also about the answer. The high value of properties in the center of many cities reveals the growing demand for this location, and also for high-density developments, because it offers the possibility of living close to work, services, and recreational and entertainment facilities. People flee to the suburbs not to escape high-density neighborhoods per se, but rather to avoid the problems that plague some parts of the inner city, where poverty, crime, and drugs are sometimes endemic. Housing preferences are not as monolithic as some imagine; many people like to live in high-rise apartments, others prefer to live in a townhouse development, and still others in single houses on a small or big lot. The dominant model of development offered to buyers now—sprawl—makes them forget that it is possible to have a house surrounded by a garden, with a lot of privacy, and still live in proximity to work, leisure, and services. This was most people's reality just a few decades ago. Most of us do not really wish to live far from work and lose so much time stuck in traffic during the commute, or take the car every time we need to buy something, or drive the children from one place to another every day because all destinations are out of reach. We got used to it, but we did not ask for it. We just assume that it had to be that way. It is that way because developers consciously limit the choices they offer—both the type of neighborhood and the mode of transportation.

A low residential density is only one aspect of sprawl; single-use environments, the absence of an activity center, and low connectivity of the road network are also part of its characteristics.[2] We used to think that low residential density is what took up so much space. We rarely considered the fact that most of the land used by sprawl is devoted to asphalt—highways, arterial roads, streets, parking lots, and driveways—rather than to the houses and yards themselves. In fact, parking lots and roads consume four times the land space required for buses, and twenty times the space necessary for railroads.[3] The use of land space—and the use of our legs—would be very different if public transportation were more prominent. A big part of land waste is also due to huge one-story buildings, such as superstores or industrial buildings, and their oversized parking lots. As Lewis Mumford wrote in his masterly history of the city, some forty years ago: "Wasteful spacing has become a substitute for intelligent civic design, far-seeing municipal organization, or rational economy."[4]

The way our living environment is now designed has a tremendous impact on our daily routine, and thereafter on our health. Let's take a look at the situation most of us have to face. But first, where did we start from?

3
A Few Steps Back…
in Human Evolution

Make your feet your friends.
— *J. M. Barrie*

July 1969, the first steps taken by humans on the moon, a striking vision for those of us who were sitting in front of the TV watching the event. It was considered one of the major technological advances of the twentieth century. There was another change, however, that had been taking place more slowly in the previous decades, unnoticed because of its apparently trivial character: walking was becoming a rare experience on earth, especially in North America.

At the beginning of the new millennium, walking is in jeopardy: people do not walk to go to work, few children walk to school, and there are fewer and fewer pedestrians on the streets. Taking the dog out is the only obligation to walk we have left, thanks to our best friend's need for its daily excursion. Otherwise, a car is required, because it is too far, too dangerous, too time-consuming or too tiring to go where we want to go on foot. So we spend more and more time sitting, not only in the car, but at work, and in front of the TV and computer as well, encouraged by a lot of modern amenities, and then wondering why so many of us get backaches. We rush outside to get things done in order to have more time sitting down passively, too exhausted to carry on any activity. Walking has been taken for granted; unfortunately, we realize its importance only when we lose the ability to do so.

Until recently, ever since we adopted the bipedal posture, walking was our main way of moving around; this fact has social and biological consequences, as well as an impact on our vision of the world. Humans are built to be able to walk and run for very long distances, without any damage other than normal fatigue. In many cultures—and not only the nomadic ones—walking is still a predominant mode of transportation. Humans were nomadic for a long period. Nomads have conquered this planet, traveling on foot from one continent to another. Even the first populations of America came here on foot via the Bering Strait. Settling down gave humans a more secure life, or should I say a more predictable one, and this is seen as progress for humankind. But to an extreme degree, a sedentary way of living—especially in permanent affluence—seems to have had disastrous consequences.

The emergence of the bipedal posture holds a predominant place in the hominization process. Preceding the increase in our brain size, the development of the ability to stand on two feet and walk took ten times longer and required many more morphological transformations. It also played a determinant role in the development of the brain, by establishing the necessary conditions for a better food regimen. In a word, human beings are characterized more by their bipedal posture than by their brain size, or even by their use of language, which appeared only later in the course of evolution.[1]

But in the space of only a few decades, we have assisted at a reversal: we have given up walking to adopt the sitting position most of the time, for locomotion, leisure, and work. To ensure that human beings would stay seated, the remote control was invented for almost everything: the garage door, the television, the car, the hi-fi system, and even the fireplace. E.T.'s magic finger acquired a new meaning I would not have thought about when I first saw the movie many years ago: it now seems it was the precursor of the remote control, the cell phone, and the computer mouse. Just the press of a finger, and you get where you want to go without changing places—a magic touch leading to obesity and impotence. I can already imagine how our great-grandchildren will look: pear-shaped, a lot heavier, with large buttocks and a big belly (because of so much sitting), a hypertrophied index finger and thumb, and muscular atrophy of the rest of the body. We have already forgotten that the human body, with so many muscles, was designed for movement and not for inaction. As reported by John Stuart Clark, an avid British cyclist: "To facilitate an independent lifestyle it is necessary to maintain an adequate level of muscle-strength, particularly in the major muscles associated with the movement of limbs."[2] Progress that fosters inaction is more like regression. The sitting human of the twenty-first century no longer resembles Rodin's "Thinker," either physically or mentally.

The bipedal posture allowed our primitive ancestors to be more vigilant about what was going on in the savannas where they lived. It was the best posture for picking fruits, watching for prey and predators, and carrying a significant amount of food in the hands rather than holding small pieces of meat between the teeth; it was also the best posture to free the hands for developing and using tools. Our ancestors had to stay alert all the time and run away when in danger. A few seconds could make a difference between life and death, or between having lunch or not, which may explain why it was preferable to stand up most of the time. Standing up makes the human body ready for action, whereas sitting is unquestionably a more passive posture. Standing up is related to vigilance. In the modern world, it does not mean vigilance toward predators, but rather against the other dangers that threaten us.

Sitting down makes us more prone to eating. I always wondered why we eat more when sitting all day, working at the computer, or traveling for a long distance by car—unless one is the driver—compared with when we go hiking or biking for hours, although sitting expends far fewer calories. I remember climbing Mount Washington in New Hampshire for hours with no desire to eat, but I can sit down hardly half a day working at the computer without being hungry. The only reason I can find is that sitting for so long constitutes an abnormally passive situation made tolerable only by ingesting more food. In many situations, the sitting position does not provide enough stimulation for our brain and senses and thus leads to eating to fill the blanks.

I have observed the same phenomenon with my pets. In summer, they spend most of their time outside chasing flies, climbing trees, watching birds, and running around, eating just when necessary because they have better things to do; but in the cold winter months, they lie down inside all day long, bored to death, incessantly begging for food. They do not get enough stimulation from their usual environment, and they are not acting as part of it, so eating becomes their main activity, their only way to be active. Fortunately for the animals, food is not as easily available to them as it is to their owners.

Playing an active role in our environment seems to limit not only the amount of time available for eating, but also the drive to eat constantly when we are not hungry. I have come to the conclusion that sitting down increases the drive for eating because it is the only way left to be active, and actively in touch with the immediate environment. If this is true, being more active would reduce the amount of ingested food, or at least the drive to eat. It might not reduce obesity, but it could help limit weight gain. In any case, it is much more difficult to eat while physically active. And even if you eat more food after being active, there is a good chance the extra calories will be burned during the next active episode. On the other hand, eating more makes us more prone to passiveness, because digestion requires all our available energy.

So what is going to happen if you stop walking and spend most of your time sitting down? What can you expect from there? *Standing up* and *sitting down:* the words themselves reveal the depth of the drama. Maybe we are at a historical turning point where sitting is a fatal issue. After spending thousands of years trying to get up, humans opted for the sitting position most of the time. Since the development of the human being repeats step by step in the course of a person's life, the evolution of other vertebrates—as shown by the similar forms of human and animal embryos in the early stages of development, or the first steps of a child, as a reminder of the onset of the upright position of our ancestors—we might wonder whether there is a link between the time spent sitting as an adult, and the future of our species as biped. Since ontogeny repeats phylogeny, maybe we are at "the end of ambulatory age," as suggested by Jane Holtz Kay.[3] What is needed now is a kind of ejector seat to take human beings out of their lethargy.

The dark side of progress is that we have become more and more secluded and inactive, with all the resulting harm to our health and social life. Many of us cannot reach most destinations on foot; children and the elderly get respiratory diseases from traffic air-pollution; obesity and its consequences threaten inactive people, as well as TV watchers and computer users; people living close to us are so unfamiliar that we feel unsafe walking around our own neighborhood; cities have become dangerous places because they were planned for cars rather than for people; pedestrians rush desperately to cross the streets, but many are killed or injured by motor vehicles while doing so; ever-greater numbers of drivers and passengers are killed or injured in car crashes; commuting to work has become a time-consuming and exhausting experience; there is less free time than ever because we spend so much time driving around frenetically; residents living close to high-speed highways endure a noisy nightmare; and we are still willing to pay to obtain all this, although we did not ask for these changes to occur. What we once thought to be a private health matter relying mainly on personal choice is now in fact a political issue—so political that the government has recently banned lawsuits blaming the food industry for people's obesity, because it could bankrupt fast-food chains and restaurants.

More and more public health experts, including the Centers for Disease Control and Prevention, now agree that the way urban neighborhoods are designed is one of the factors responsible for physical inactivity, and the resulting epidemic of obesity and its health consequences in the American population.[4-6] In September 2003, two scientific journals—the *American Journal of Public Health* and the *American Journal of Health Promotion*—devoted entire issues to this subject. Specialists now talk about "obesogenic" environments, that is, environments designed in such a way that they lead to obesity because of the unlimited availability of high-calorie food and a lifestyle encouraging or even forcing physical inactivity.[7]

In December 2003, *Newsweek* magazine reviewed the top ten challenges in health and medicine; not surprisingly, obesity stood first as the biggest health crisis facing the country, and it was stated that its cure would require changes in our lifestyle.[8] Every week, the press reports new adverse consequences of the situation we are now facing.

The American Medical Association (AMA) has attributed the obesity epidemic not only to eating more, but also to the decreasing opportunities in daily life to burn energy; it says helping people get back to walking or bicycling should be a first target in fighting the epidemic.[9] The AMA observes, "The most effective solutions to the obesity epidemic are likely environmental. . . . Restoration of physical activity as part of the daily routine represents a critical goal."[10]

Human effort, not so long ago associated with hard work and low-status jobs, is not valued any more, unless there is no other purpose than fitness. Walking for transport, climbing the stairs when there is an escalator, opening a can of soup or a garage door without any electric or automatic device, turning on television or music without the remote control—all those now seem nonsense, if not awkward. Those who do not comply with this passive way of living look suspicious, marginal, or even stupid. According to Ian Roberts, the Australian author of *Pedalling Health*, "Saving energy in the form of human effort appears to have become a cultural norm."[11]

For our primitive ancestors, saving energy may have been a necessary requirement for survival, but only for short periods, when food was scarce or some danger imminent. These ancestors could not have been fat, because they would have been unable to run. Being slim was a must. In fact, wild animals are rarely fat, not because they do not eat enough, but rather so

A TWO-YEAR
OBESITY NEWS CALENDAR

Almost every day, there is some news warning us about the obesity epidemic and its adverse consequences. Here are some examples illustrating the growing importance of the problem in the news over the last two years.[12]

2003

JAN	Obesity "a Threat" to U.S. Security
FEB	Watch Those Cookies
MAR	Risk of Excess Weight Increases in Unsafe Neighborhoods
APR	Prolonged TV Watching Increases Obesity and Diabetes Risk
MAY	Birth Defects Linked to Obesity
JUNE	Western-Style Consumption Worldwide Fuels "Globesity"
JULY	Hungry but Fat
AUG	Obesity Goes Global
SEPT	As Weight Goes Up, Life Span Goes Down
OCT	Extreme Obesity Ballooning in U.S. Adults
NOV	US Kids Show Early Signs of Heart Disease
DEC	Pets Mirror Nation's Obesity Problem

2004

JAN	Taxes Pay for Most Obesity Costs
FEB	Obesity Is the New Tobacco
MAR	We're Eating Ourselves to Death
APR	Schools That Can Soda Cut Obesity
MAY	Three-Year-Old Dies from Obesity
JUNE	Obesity Straining Health Care System
JULY	Sedentary Behaviors Are Linked to Childhood Obesity
AUG	Obesity Ups Cancer Risk
SEPT	Obese Trauma Patients More Likely to Die of Their Injuries
OCT	Longer Commutes Lead to Wider Waistlines
NOV	Fat Americans Costing Airlines More on Fuel
DEC	Emigrating to America Makes You Fat

they can run away from predators, chase their own food, and travel long distances. They have to be on the move constantly. In nature, normal weight is not a matter of beauty but a survival necessity, and it works the same way for human beings as it does for other animals. Just think how much more difficult it is to climb stairs carrying ten additional pounds, and then try to imagine how hard it can be if you are 100 pounds overweight, which is now the case for at least four million American adults.[13] A flock of overweight spring warblers trying to travel thousands of miles twice a year to reach their summer or winter habitat would seem ridiculous to us; the birds would have little chance of reaching their destination. How can we find it acceptable for humans?

Saving energy is no longer necessary; it has never been necessary in the long run, and, in fact, it clearly appears rather dangerous. Humans do not have to strive any longer to survive. The availability of food makes any attempt to store it in our own bodies useless. We are reaching a turning point where we may soon have to spend a lot more energy to survive.

There is actually an energy crisis, but this time, the problem is a surplus of human energy, the amount we store, not allowing the body to spend it in our daily life routine. As noted by nutrition expert James Hill of the University of Colorado in Denver, *there is a mismatch between our genes and the environment:* "Our ancestors had to expend a lot of energy just to get through the day. So, our genes say 'Eat when food is available, and rest when you don't have to be active.' But now food is always available, and technology has made it easy to be sedentary. So it's really the environment that's causing the problem."[14]

For millions of years, when food scarcity was the rule, eating was a survival behavior, so the brain still reacts to promote eating, despite the fact that we are constantly surrounded by food, especially high-calorie food packed with fat and sugar. Our brain tells us to eat, in case there is a shortage in the near future, as there often was before. But due to phenomenal advances in the agriculture and food industries, our environment has changed; in only a few decades, we have become overwhelmed by a surfeit of food. Unfortunately, the behavioral adaptation to this new reality has not yet been achieved. Worse, we simultaneously fell for an extremely low-energy lifestyle. Overeating could even be seen as a suicide attempt, a self-destructive habit for an extremely sedentary and affluent civilization.

Very often, we bless modern technology for making our lives easier without realizing that it has also made us extremely lazy, and not really conscious of the negative consequences of this induced inactivity. Few of us do strenuous work. Transportation does not require human energy any more. Even for walking, new technological inventions tend to reduce the amount of human energy expenditure: in Hong Kong, for example, a half-mile-long horizontal escalator, known as a travelator, crossing the city has brought residents close to their work every day since 1994. In North America, some golf courses now have travelators for deep-slope areas.

Our modern lifestyle has relegated physical activity to our leisure time, and thus to individual willpower. We now have to make a decision to exercise, since it is no longer part of our daily routine. However, it does not seem to be the right answer to this new societal problem. The environment of our species has been modified so much that relying mainly on an individual solution to bring back a healthy lifestyle has little chance of working. According to Leonard Epstein, a specialist in childhood obesity at Stanford University, reducing sedentary behavior may be more important than promoting physical activity itself.[15]

The best way to increase the level of exercise in the population is to make it part of the daily routine, so one does not even have to think about performing any kind of physical activity. The key to success is to exercise without realizing it, as did our ancestors. They never told themselves, We have to exercise to stay fit or to lose weight. They just did, because there was no other choice, because it was the normal way of doing things. They had to use their legs to go somewhere, sometimes for quite long distances, and often faster than we are doing now with cars.

Strangely, we do not question the choices others have made for us, leaving me with the feeling that we are already too passive to react. Although we like to think we are the planners of our own lifestyle, other forces are in

A WALK AROUND THE WORLD

The enormous endurance of the human body for walking is well illustrated by the journey of Polly Letofsky, the first American woman to walk around the world. The purpose of her trip was to raise awareness about breast cancer. Leaving her hometown of Vail, Colorado, with her rolling backpack, the forty-two-year-old woman crossed twenty-two countries on foot in five years, walking 14,000 miles for 1,825 consecutive days before returning home at the end of July 2004 (see walking.about.com).

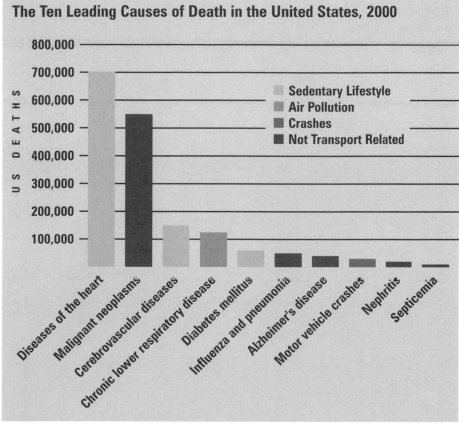

The Ten Leading Causes of Death in the United States, 2000

Todd Litman, 2004

fact deciding for us. And we witness these changes, trying to adapt, and thinking it is the only possible avenue. This state of passiveness and docility as the result of a narrowing of our external world, reinforced by the widespread usage of the private car and its consequences, was already pointed out forty years ago by Lewis Mumford in his book *The City in History*, in a section devoted to the suburban type of development, which was then only at its beginning.[16]

Walk for Your Life describes in more detail the causes and negative consequences of giving up walking as a means of circulation, and of restricting ourselves to the sitting position for most of our activities of daily life, whether it is work, leisure, or transportation. The emphasis is on the social and health consequences of walking less, although many other aspects of our lives may also be impaired. Finally, possible adjustments are considered—personal as well as collective—that could improve our quality of life and our health.

4

Trying to Walk
in the United States

We live in a fast-paced society. Walking slows us down.
—*Robert Sweetgall*

After many trips to European countries, where I used to travel on
foot, by train, or by bus, three years ago I decided to get away
from my snowy home town and go to Florida to enjoy the mild
weather of April. Fort Lauderdale was the destination, and a motel about
a mile and a half from the beach seemed a good choice, because it would
give me the opportunity to walk. Driving to the beach for such a short distance seemed ridiculous to me, so I did not rent a car. After a very cold
winter spent mostly inside, I desperately needed outdoor exercise.

To my disappointment, the only pedestrians on the streets were hobos
digging into the garbage. Car drivers honked and yelled at me as if I were
some kind of strange person, or maybe a prostitute, but surely my walking
activity did not look normal to them. Walking is now perceived as a sign of
low status, because people who can afford to own a car do not walk. In fact,
it is well known that low-income people walk more than those in other income groups. This negative perception could even prevent some people
from walking, to avoid looking powerless or poor.

So many cars passing, seeming to go nowhere endlessly. I wondered what
the purpose of this ceaseless agitation was. I felt rather insecure realizing that
nobody walked to go anywhere, despite the perfect weather, the proximity
of destinations, and the availability of sidewalks. I was even told not to walk

to the restaurant—only a short distance from the motel—after dark because it could be dangerous; so I went to eat early and noticed that all the other clients had arrived in their cars. I then realized it was impossible to behave as I did in Europe, or even in my own town. So after three days I changed my airplane ticket and went back home with my pedestrian dream.

A few years before that incident, I was in one of the beach cities just south of Los Angeles. A great place for pedestrians, since the weather is perfect most of the time and the beach is within walking distance, along with stores and other commodities. I was surprised to notice how empty the streets were, except for a few joggers. I realized that walking was not fashionable at all, and I wondered if a pedestrian could be viewed as anything other than too poor to own a car. Sure, there were a lot of people outside; but they were concentrated on the paved path along the ocean, biking, jogging, or roller-skating. Those who wanted to exercise ran away from the streets, even if it was safe and quiet in the area. Nobody was trying to reach any specific destination on foot. Utilitarian walking did not exist any more; the residents had already conceded the streets to cars. No one stood outside, looking at other people passing by. Despite the weather, there were no sidewalk cafés just to gather around with friends or neighbors. Americans have gone to the moon, but they have not yet taken possession of their own streets. Walking has become a recreational activity rather than a way of getting around.

I wondered then why the streets of many American cities were so empty, but I now had the answer. The widespread use of the car has fostered a kind of development incompatible with pedestrian life, and this human invention has changed our behavior, individually and as a society. As a creature of human beings, the car has become almost a species in itself, the way it freely moves around and conquers more than its share of the available space, relying on nonrenewable resources to assure its own survival. And as we compete for the same ecological niche, we are losing the battle against it. It has made our walkable habitat shrink constantly, with the same result as for endangered species. As will be shown later, the decrease in walking and in physical activity as a whole, as well as the tremendous rise in obesity, are the most obvious symptoms of our defeat by the automobile and the kind of development it has brought with it.

Walking has even become somewhat suspicious. *The New York Times* recently reported on New Yorkers who, trying with difficulty to walk in Los Angeles as they would do at home, were struck by the emptiness of the sidewalks; according to one would-be pedestrian, "motorists are staring at you as though you have suddenly grown a second head or split the seat of your pants."[1] It is well known that people from New York walk more than residents from all other cities, due to their compact, mixed-use environment, and to the availability of public transit. The author of this article recalled a science fiction story called "The Pedestrian," written by Ray Bradbury at the beginning of the fifties, about a man who enjoyed walking the vacant streets after dark and was taken to a mental institution for doing so rather than staying home watching television. Bradbury set his story in the year 2052, but it seems as if we are almost there.

TWENTY-ONE STEPS FOR SMART WALKING

1 **CHOOSE THE RIGHT SHOES.** They can be leather shoes or running shoes; it does not matter. They have to breathe and be flexible and not too tight. They do not have to be expensive, but they should be very comfortable right away. Walking should not be a painful experience. Pay as much attention to your shoes as to the tires of your car. Your feet are precious, and you should pamper them.

2 **CONVINCE YOURSELF YOU HAVE ENOUGH TIME.** This is probably the most difficult step. You believe you are so busy you don't have time to exercise. But try to estimate how much time you spend sitting after meals or in front of the television, and transfer thirty of those minutes to your walking activity.

3 **ESTABLISH A ROUTINE.** A new habit always requires discipline. A good way to get it is to develop a routine. Try to walk at a specific time of the day: before or after meals, or on your way to work or to go shopping. It will be easier if it fits in your daily schedule.

4 **DEFINE A SET OF ROUTES.** If you expect to walk two, three, or four miles in a row, use your car first to set up the best routes and measure the distance. Then choose between the selected routes according to the distance you want to travel on that specific day.

5 **WALK SAFE.** Use sidewalks where available. Otherwise, walk facing road traffic. Avoid high-traffic roads and streets with blind walls. At night, choose streets with good lighting and wear bright colors. Do not walk after drinking too much alcohol. It increases your risk of an accident.

6 **SET A GOAL AND STICK TO IT.** Be realistic. If you set your goal too high at first, you may have not enough discipline to maintain your schedule. Try to set a goal for a day. But a weekly goal would be better if some days are really too busy.

7 **CHECK DESTINATIONS A MILE OR LESS AWAY.** It can be your workplace, a store, a coffee shop, a park, or a friend's house. It is often easier to go for a walk when you have a purpose. If a store is reachable on foot, buy a little at a time and go more often.

8 **FIND A PARTNER.** If you do not feel safe or lack motivation to walk alone, find someone to walk with you, human or canine. You will enjoy the walk more and probably go further than you would have alone.

9 **DON'T BOTHER WITH THE WEATHER.** Do not use the weather as an excuse for not walking, unless it is really too hot. Just dress appropriately. What may look like bad weather from inside is often much better once you are out.

10 **SEE YOURSELF AS PART OF YOUR ENVIRONMENT.** Just enjoy looking around instead of feeling threatened by what you think might be an inhospitable environment. There may be nice people around, or trees and birds you don't know yet. In my sister's neighborhood, an Ottawa suburb, I was filled with wonder when I saw rabbits running around freely.

11 **GET FREE OF YOUR REMOTE CONTROL.** These devices make you fat and lazy. They prevent you from burning calories. Instead, walk to the TV set to change channels, and to the garage door to open it.

12 **CHECK YOUR WEIGHT DAILY.** If you are a little heavier than the day before, walk more (and eat less). This is not an obsession but a weight-control routine that prevents the insidious accumulation of fat in your body. Better to prevent overweight early.

13 **WEAR A PEDOMETER.** If you are the type of person who likes to measure everything, wearing a pedometer will give you the count of steps you made on your trip and the distance you traveled; some models even provide the number of calories you burned. This way, you will be able to check your progress.

14 **GET A WALKING STICK.** If you limit your walking activity because you are afraid of dogs, carry a walking stick. You may not have to use it, but it can act as a good deterrent and give you more self-confidence. It may even prevent falls among older walkers.

15 **PARK AND WALK.** Park as far away as you can when going to the shopping mall. Parking too close to the entrance increases the risk your car will be hit by another car, and your own risk of getting less fit and fatter.

16 **GET OFF THE BUS/TRAIN ONE STATION AHEAD.** If you take public transit to work, don't stop too close to the office. You will sit down all day anyway. There will be plenty of time to rest. Spend some physical energy so you will have more mental energy.

17 WEAR A WALKMAN. If despite your efforts the trip seems too dull or the area too noisy, bring a Walkman or a portable radio so you can listen to music or news as you walk.

18 WALK YOUR CHILDREN TO SCHOOL. If your children's school is within walking distance, walk them to school instead of driving them. The walking habit has to be learned early to stay effective later. Don't forget that less driving around the school means a safer route for children walking. And both you and your children will benefit from walking together.

19 JOIN A WALKING CLUB. If your motivation is directly related to the number of people walking with you, or if you cannot find a partner to walk with, join a walking club. They are numerous in the United States, and they offer a lot of excursions. It is also a good opportunity to meet other people with the same goals.

20 WALK FOR PLEASURE. You should not walk only to get fit or to lose weight. Walking is not a medication. You can do it just for fun too. Unless you enjoy it, it will not be part of your normal life, and the habit may not last long.

21 ALWAYS REMEMBER THAT WALKING IS A SURVIVAL NECESSITY. The human body was designed for walking. This activity may help you control your weight, stay fit and independent, and keep you in touch with—and in control of—your environment. Neither terrorist attacks nor crime are as dangerous as the threats of obesity and road carnage. You may need your legs, so exercise them before it is too late.

5

The Value of Walking,
and the Price of Not Walking

Walking takes longer... than any other known form
of locomotion except crawling. Thus it stretches time and prolongs life.
Life is already too short to waste on speed.
—*Edward Abbey*

We like to think we live in a very efficient society, but when it comes to transportation, this is not so evident. Even for very small distances, we use the car when we could get there just as easily on foot or by bike. By doing so, we contribute to traffic congestion, and it often takes more time than walking to reach the destination. We also deprive ourselves of good opportunities for social contacts with fellow citizens met on the road. Relying on motor-vehicle driving for most of our trips contributes not only to traffic congestion, but also to increased road injuries and fatalities, air pollution, soil erosion, land waste, and wildlife habitat destruction; it has a dramatic impact on climatic change and accentuates global warming, and so on. The costs associated with these consequences are extremely high. Reliance on automobiles has led to the construction of huge parking lots where it can be difficult to find a place at specific hours of the day, or for some days of the year, and which are left completely deserted at other times. The words of Lewis Mumford are still useful here: "Speed in locomotion should be a function of human purpose.... What an effective network requires is the largest number of alternative modes of transportation, at varying speeds and volumes, for different functions and purposes."[1]

This simple statement should be memorized by urban planners and

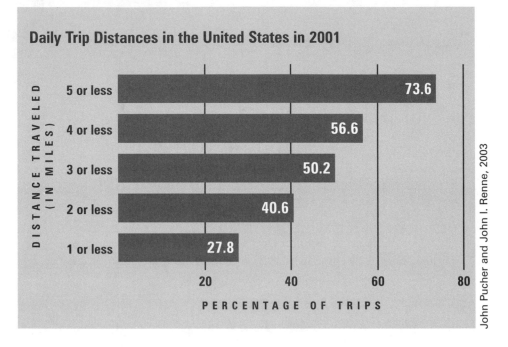

Daily Trip Distances in the United States in 2001

DISTANCE TRAVELED (IN MILES)

5 or less — 73.6
4 or less — 56.6
3 or less — 50.2
2 or less — 40.6
1 or less — 27.8

PERCENTAGE OF TRIPS

20 40 60 80

John Pucher and John I. Renne, 2003

municipal authorities, because it is at the basis of a livable and healthy city. Utilitarian walking has to find its place among other modes of transportation, and promoting its usage can even make driving a more pleasant and efficient experience. It has nothing to do with giving up automobiles, but rather with favoring walking for short-distance trips and cars or mass transit for longer ones.

For a short distance, the fastest way to move around is often on foot or by bike, especially when a lot of people are moving at the same time, creating congestion on the roads. An experiment carried out in Montreal in 2004 showed that a distance of nearly five miles was covered faster by bike than by car at rush hour, at a cost six times less.[2] Commuting to my job takes between fifteen and thirty minutes by car, although the distance—three miles—is very short. At best, my average speed is twelve miles per hour. There are exactly sixteen red lights on my way. Sometimes I spend more time waiting for them to turn green than driving—burning gasoline instead of human energy. If there were less traffic at rush hour, I would be able to travel by bike and reach my destination in less time, following quieter streets. But there are no showers at work. It is very easy to understand that for such a short distance, the car is not the most efficient mode of transportation. Nevertheless, most workers have to stick with it, because there are not enough facilities available to do otherwise. No showers at work, no bicycle racks, no public transit.

The paradox revealed by Ivan Illich in his 1974 book *Energy and Equity* is illustrated by the fact that beyond a critical level, speed does not save any further time but rather induces a shortage, so the motor vehicle itself creates distances.[3] As Marshall McLuhan said some forty years ago, technology extends the range of the human body and mind, but these extensions also result in amputations, which are the hidden consequences of technology and the counterpart of the extensions. Fascinated and obsessed with these extensions, we choose to ignore or minimize the amputations at our own peril. Often the adverse consequences of these extensions outweigh their benefits. We voluntarily choose to accept the disadvantages of technology because we worship the privileges given by the extensions; "The extension of the automobile amputates the need for a highly developed walking culture," and this leads to a more sedentary lifestyle and to obesity.[4]

More recently, Todd Litman of the Victoria Transport Policy Institute in Victoria, British Columbia, has studied the economic value of walkability and showed how improved walkability increases accessibility, provides consumer and public cost savings, increases community livability, improves public health, and supports strategic economic development, land use, and equity objectives.[5]

In her brilliant history of walking, Rebecca Solnit draws an analogy between walking activity and an indicator species, one that characterizes the health of an ecosystem. "Its endangerment or diminishment can be an early warning sign of systemic trouble," she observes.[6] By reducing the places we can walk, the human habitat shrinks, and we confine ourselves to the private sphere. If this is the case, the gym could be seen as a kind of wildlife preserve for physical exertion: "A preserve protects species whose habitat is vanishing elsewhere, and the gym accommodates the survival of bodies after the abandonment of the original sites of bodily exertion. The gym is the interior space that compensates for the disappearance of outside and a stopgap measure in the erosion of the bodies."[7]

The human scale of our habitat is disappearing, and human behavior is such that we now drive to the gym, trying to park as close as possible to the entrance, in order to spend our energy walking on a treadmill. In the gym, the treadmill, by simulating walking, suggests that the outside space has disappeared. Of this perverse device, Solnit observes, "Walking activity has reduced itself to the alternate movement of the lower limbs, losing all its other functions."[8]

Sometimes in my car I feel safe, as if I were on safari, with the dangerous animals outside and me well protected inside my steel-and-glass bubble. Thinking twice, I have concluded that the animals are not outside, threatening us: rather, we are in their womb. They have swallowed us, and we now live inside them, like Jonah in the whale. We spend a huge part of our income to buy them, provide them with food and shelter, and keep them in good condition. Even their short lifespan makes us their slaves, because we have to get a new one after only a few years. Cars isolate human beings from each other. They kill some of us randomly. They have become the masters of this world, and we still fervently pretend they have brought more freedom into our lives.

6

The Conspiracy

If I could not walk far and fast,
I think I should just explode and perish.
—Charles Dickens

In my biology classes in high school and college, I learned that in the animal kingdom, big animals usually eat smaller ones; this is especially evident among fish. But in the human species, the reverse seems true. Reading magazines and newspapers and watching the news on television is enough to make you realize that those who really profit from our secluded and sedentary way of life and its consequences on our waistlines and health are more likely to be thin than obese. Those who make the rules, who design roads and suburban developments, who own television networks, food or car companies, and junk-food restaurants, and even those who help obese people lose weight, look better, and improve their health, are conspicuously less fat than the rest of us. Wealthier people are usually thinner. It happens that they also have a bigger role in deciding how this world is going to be shaped and run.

Someone must be profiting from this situation, otherwise it would not exist. On one side, there are industries that make people more sedentary and fat, confining them to the house, the car, or the television or computer screen. On the other side, the fight against obesity and sedentary life has also become a good source of profit. From dieting products, extra-extra-large clothing, miracle slimming drugs, health counseling, surgery, and larger coffins, a lot of people are making good money taking care of the fattest ones. The slimming business itself was worth $40 billion in the United States in 2003.[1]

Beyond profits, there is also the social fragmentation created by a more secluded way of life, which increases our passive willingness to follow the rules dictated by powerful individuals, even though doing may not be to our benefit. Ordinary citizens are caught between the two markets, not realizing to what extent they are the targets of these big businesses that tell people they have the right to decide what is good for them, and that having a choice allows people to use their freedom. Unhealthy eating habits and physical inactivity are then seen as resulting from personal misbehavior, rather than from our social environment. But when two thirds of the American population is overweight or obese, it is difficult to put the blame on the individual. As Walker Poston, a nutrition specialist from the Baylor College of Medicine in Houston, Texas, wrote in 1999: "Obesity is an environmental issue. . . . Obesity-promoting behaviors are controlled by factors outside the individual and obese individuals cannot be expected to have total self-control over their weight in an environment that promotes weight gain by reinforcing overeating and inactivity any more than they can control their genes."[2]

In fact, there is no real choice. Here are the options:

■ *A secluded life in neighborhoods where residents cannot interact much with each other,* because there are no public places for doing so, and few opportunities for casual contacts with others, where people cannot send their children to school on foot, cannot walk to work, stores, or other facilities because they are out of reach, and cannot cross the street because it is too dangerous. A place where everyone feels unsafe going on foot when it is deserted—which is most of the time, because single-use environments are the rule, so only one function is present at a time, work, stores, or residences—so better to use the car. A place where everyone sits passively in front of the television at night, watching the lives of other people, fictional or real, instead of living their own lives. This individualistic lifestyle, where citizens are more and more isolated from each other, profits those who shape this world and make decisions for us. These decisions have led to huge profits for a small number.

■ *A situation where a high proportion of household income goes to transportation,* especially in suburban areas where a car is a necessity; and in which the poorer you are, the higher the proportion, making it almost impossible to save enough money to buy a decent house or create wealth. Car dependence is the rule: you are out of luck if you are too young, too old, or too poor to drive. Too bad also for those who spend hours every week stuck in traffic while commuting to work. Too bad for the numerous people who are killed, injured, or permanently handicapped in traffic accidents. According to the environmentalist Andrew Kimbrell, ninety million Americans have sustained disabling injuries in car accidents (see www.newurbanism.org). There is a business that profits from taking care of them too.

■ *A world where schools are located in a no-man's-land away from residential areas*, as if they were industrial plants—and they even look like it—and where children cannot walk because it is too far, or bike because it is too dangerous. Facing a lack of public funding, these schools reduce the amount of time devoted to physical education, while signing exclusivity contracts with vending companies that place machines packed with snack foods and soft drinks in the cafeteria, thus encouraging physical inactivity and unhealthy food habits among generations of children, and preparing them for a lifetime of serious medical problems.

■ *An urban environment so unfriendly to pedestrians that it is almost impossible to go out for a walk* and spend the surplus of energy from a high-calorie meal, an oversize portion of processed food ingested because we were too tired or too busy to cook. After a while, the ultimate solutions to this weight gain are dieting, liposuction, or stomach stapling.

■ *A lifestyle in which sidewalk window-shopping has been replaced by walking inside shopping centers*—leading to the disappearance of the public realm—and thereafter by driving for short distances between superstores surrounded by a sea of asphalt, thus restraining pedestrian movement as much as possible. To the loss of a sense of community is added the loss of exercise as part of daily life.

■ *An environment in which it is increasingly difficult to exercise in the normal course of daily life* because so many technological devices promote physical inactivity, while at the same time we are exposed to plenty of cheap food and encouraged to eat as much as we can; the Sunday brunch has very perverse consequences. The *raison d'être* of remote controls can be seen from different perspectives. The ability to control things from a distance allows us to save energy while giving us a sense of power; but is it really necessary to save energy? It seems as though we do not spend enough. Remote controls are also—and mainly—new ways to make profits for those who design, produce, sell, and repair these devices. This is what we call progress.

■ *A living space where children get asthma from breathing polluted air*, especially if they are poor, because they are more likely to live in a low-rent apartment near high-traffic roads and highways.

Many of these decisions seem to be made by a few wealthy and powerful corporate groups based on narrow self-interest and greed rather than on community welfare. The net effect of these self-serving decisions is an insufficient level of physical activity for the general populace in an environment that discourages activity, exacerbated by a lot of unnecessary technological devices, a food supply system that overfeeds and over-fattens people, and a weight-control industry that gorges itself on the false hopes of those who want to become attractively slim again. Our socioeconomic system instills and reinforces these destructive habits early in childhood so that they become deeply rooted. Consequently, the habits become irreversible for most, as the wheels of power and fortune continue to turn. To say the least, this not a system "promoting the general welfare" that the writers of the U.S. Constitution might have endorsed.

Part 2

Urban Sprawl
and Car Dependence

7

Underestimating the Problem: The Victims

The only way you run into someone else in L.A. is in a car crash.
—*Susan Sarandon, on why she moved to New York City*

TRAFFIC FATALITIES

Between 1970 and 1995, 1.2 million people died on America's roads, nearly 50,000 a year,[1] but we rarely hear about this carnage. It seems very hard to believe. Other deaths get much more attention than road fatalities. Closer to the present and in a shorter time, during the first seven months of the SARS (severe acute respiratory syndrome) epidemic of 2003, 728 people died worldwide from the disease, and the media talked extensively about the problem every day. In the same period, 583,000 people died in motor-vehicle accidents around the world, but it went almost unnoticed.[2] The road is the main source of violent death.

Despite our perceptions, traffic fatalities are much more important than homicides in the United States. Traffic fatalities were 2.7 times more frequent than homicides in 2001: in that year alone, there were 41,821 deaths on the road, versus 15,517 deaths by homicide. The ratio has increased considerably since 1991, making motor-vehicle accidents the greatest danger people face when they leave their homes.[3] Murders are much more widely publicized than motor-vehicle fatalities, however, and people are more concerned about crime than road accidents when going out, even though the victims of violent assaults usually know their aggressors. Being in a car gives a false sense of safety, and of power as well. But this invincibility is only apparent, as revealed by the numbers.

We are so used to people dying on the roads that we consider it only as a very sad but inevitable part of life, a kind of bad luck for those involved. We grieve, and we forget. Although these deaths do not happen on purpose, they are not accidental at all. They happen because we tolerate a model of technological and urban development that makes them not only possible but likely.

THE EMERGENCE OF SPRAWL

During the second half of the twentieth century, road engineers, car companies, city planners, local authorities, zoning laws, and superstore owners all contributed to an automobile-oriented development largely incompatible with walking. In many cities, we helped cut back the public transportation system, thus reducing even more the possibility of walking. So it is not surprising that three quarters of Americans say their day-to-day tasks would be more difficult without a car, and 91 percent mention their car as an important aspect of their freedom.[4] One of the reasons the automobile seems to embody freedom is that the kind of urban development now prevailing makes people prisoners of the built environment: prisoners at home, at work, or shopping. Most of the time, the only way to escape from one of these areas is by car. The car frees us from the prison created by a car-oriented environment. In a pedestrian-friendly environment, the car would not be such a symbol of freedom.

The low-density type of development promoted during the second half of the twentieth century made public transportation a much less viable option than driving. At the same time, reliance on the automobile encouraged by sprawl had a huge impact on many aspects of our health and social life and on the environment as well. When the automobile is the only available means of circulation, it makes an area as vulnerable as a town whose economy relies on a single employer. If an unusual or catastrophic event disrupts the normal course of things, there is no alternative basis for the town's economy that would allow the town to avoid collapse. Many once-thriving mining towns, for example, became ghost towns after the mines shut down.

The idea that urban sprawl has an impact, not only on transportation or the environment but on our health as well, is gaining ground. As urban sprawl is characterized by low-density development and separated land uses, it is directly related to car usage. Destinations are too far to be reached on foot. Most of the time, this means we need to have two cars instead of one, and possibly even three or four, when the kids get older. Air pollution resulting from this kind of development is already a known cause of respiratory problems, but now public health experts blame physical inactivity, and the resulting obesity epidemic, at least partly on this type of urban design. Urban sprawl has recently been found to be associated with obesity and hypertension; a study involving more than 200,000 adults from 448 American counties and eighty-three metropolitan areas showed that people living in more sprawling counties weighed more and had a greater prevalence of high blood pressure than residents of more compact counties.[5] These people weigh more whether or not they walk for exercise during their leisure time, suggesting they probably miss the health benefits of walking as part of their daily routine; urban form was more important in explaining overweight than leisure-time walking.[6]

Previous research carried out for Smart Growth America found that people living in more sprawling areas tend to drive greater distances, own more cars, breathe more polluted air because of the higher ozone concentration, face a greater risk of traffic fatalities, and walk and use transit less. The number of cars per household was also higher in more sprawling areas; according to the authors of the study, the average household vehicle ownership is an indicator of how dependent a population is on the automobile for basic transportation.[7] Data from the National Personal Transportation Survey indicate that residents from higher-density urban areas make about 25 percent fewer car trips and more than twice as many pedestrian and transit trips than the national average.[8] In the San Francisco Bay area, the number of total daily trips—as well as car trips—made by residents of suburban areas was found to be higher than for residents of traditional neighborhoods, while overall transit use in the traditional areas was about more than double the rate in suburban areas; moreover, pedestrian activity was 50 percent higher in traditional communities.[9]

It even seems that people living in more dense older cities—which does not necessarily mean inner cities—are now better off, because they do not get stuck in traffic; they have easier access to parks and to a wide selection of stores; they can walk or take public transit to work; and their children can walk to school. They can get from one place to another on foot, so walking is not just a recreational activity for them. Central business districts are particularly suited for pedestrians because driving can be difficult and inefficient over short distances due to the high level of traffic and the difficulty of finding a place to park. These two factors act as deterrents to driving and thereby promote walking as the quickest way to get to a destination. This convenience disappears in lower-density areas such as the suburbs.

Although many people moved to the suburbs for a better quality of life and to escape inner-city problems, the newer suburbs do not provide the elements that made the older suburbs appealing. According to a survey of new-home buyers cited by the American Medical Association, almost all the amenities that made communities desirable places to live were those that promoted physical activity, such as walking and jogging trails, outdoor swimming pools, playgrounds, and parks.[10]

How can we expect people to walk when there are no sidewalks in the neighborhood, no shops or other commodities to walk to, no workplace or school or entertainment at walking distance? Even many parking lots have become unsafe because they are so large they encourage drivers to speed through them. We have created a world where walking is not only unnecessary but almost impossible and even dangerous. In this context, one has to decide to walk, mainly for exercise, but those who are willing to do so are probably already more concerned about fitness than others and more prone to take action to keep in shape. So many of us do not move enough to stay fit and healthy.

PEDESTRIAN MAYHEM

Every year, nearly 5,000 pedestrians are killed by motor vehicles in the United States, a higher toll than in the collapse of the World Trade Center.[11] These are lonely and anonymous deaths, however, so anonymous that we do not even realize how big the problem is. These people were just crossing the street, walking to school, or waiting at a bus stop. They were not practicing any kind of dangerous sport. They were just walking. According to the Surface Transportation Policy Project, 78,000 more pedestrians are injured in traffic crashes every year; many are disabled for life. And this number represents only the reported accidents. Some people are hit by cars but do not call the police or visit the hospital because they do not consider the damage to be serious enough, or because they have no health insurance, or for other reasons.

The most dangerous places to walk are metropolitan areas marked by newer low-density developments with wide, high-speed arterials offering few pedestrian facilities such as sidewalks and crosswalks. Nearly half of pedestrian deaths occur where no crosswalk is available.

While streets are getting wider and wider, pedestrian lights are too short to allow people to cross easily and safely. These lights are timed for young adults in good condition and do not give elderly people enough time to cross. So the elderly are at a greater risk of getting killed by a car. Although the elderly account for 13 percent of the population, they represent 22 percent of pedestrian fatalities.[12]

The pedestrian fatality rate varies widely according to the geographic area. The ten areas with the highest pedestrian fatality rates are located in the South or Southwest, five of them in Florida (Orlando, Tampa-St. Petersburg-Clearwater, West Palm Beach-Boca Raton, Miami-Fort Lauderdale, and Jacksonville).[13] Interestingly, even though New York has the highest proportion of people walking to work, it has one of the lowest pedestrian fatality rates in the country; it is also the most compact metropolitan area. Lower annual fatality rates are usually found in denser cities such as Portland (Oregon), New York, Chicago, and Philadelphia, while higher rates are mainly found in low-density cities such as Dallas, Atlanta, Phoenix, and Tampa.[14]

Ethnic and racial minorities are overrepresented in pedestrian deaths: African-Americans account for one of five deaths, although they represent only 12 percent of the population. Latino pedestrians are also slightly overrepresented. These people are less likely to own a car and more likely to walk, increasing their exposure to traffic; a higher proportion of minority people walk to work than whites.[15]

Pedestrian fatality rates are much higher in the United States than in other industrialized countries, although we walk less. The U.S. rate is fourteen times higher than that of Germany or the Netherlands.[16] In Europe and Japan, 20 to 50 percent of all trips are still made on foot, and bike trips are also much more common. In a literature review of the relationship between physical activity and the built environment, the Centers for Disease Control and Prevention (CDC) reported that in Sweden in 1990, 39 percent of all trips were made on foot, compared to 36 percent by car. In other countries such as Austria, Denmark, Italy, the Netherlands, and Switzerland, in 2000 the percentage of trips made on foot or by bike was equal to or greater than the proportion of trips made by car.[17]

Although the pedestrian fatality rate has decreased over the last decades, the concomitant decline in walking suggests that the decrease in the fatality rate results mainly from a lower exposure to traffic. Fewer pedestrians get killed because there are fewer pedestrians on the roads.

CHILDREN: AN ENDANGERED SPECIES

Children rely more heavily than adults on walking to move around and go places, making them especially at risk for traffic accidents, because their exposure is higher than that of any other age group. The risk of injury among children has been strongly associated with traffic volume[18-22] and high density of curb parking.[23-25] The proportion of vehicles exceeding the speed limit was also a factor related to injuries.[26,27]

Child pedestrian death rates have fallen in many countries over the past two decades, but according to some experts, the statistic only reflects the decline in children's traffic exposure:[28] because parents consider the streets too dangerous, they do not let their children play outside without supervision, and they drive them almost everywhere they have to go. The rare initiatives aimed at reducing the level of traffic were also found to have a positive impact on child pedestrian death rates; in New Zealand, for example, government policies to reduce car usage following the energy crisis in the 1970s resulted in a strong reduction in the child pedestrian mortality rate.[29]

When there is no play area adjacent to the home, the risk of child pedestrian injuries is five times higher than usual,[30] which may explain why children from multifamily residential areas are more prone to traffic accidents.[31] The explanation given is that in both these situations, a child might be more likely to use the street, driveway, or parking lot as the main play area, thereby increasing the chance for contact with motor vehicles.[32] In Montreal, one study showed that most accidents involving child pedestrians occurred between May and August, usually on weekdays and during the late afternoon. Most of these accidents happened on straight sections of streets, far from traffic signals, and under good conditions of visibility; according to the authors, cars parked in school areas also represented a danger.[33]

Last year, on my own street, I realized how dangerous the environment was for a young cyclist, even in a relatively quiet area. On a street with no sidewalks, a seven-year-old boy on a bike suddenly materialized in front of my car as he emerged from behind a minivan. Fortunately, I was driving slowly enough to be able to stop almost instantly. There were so many cars parked on that side of the street that it was impossible to see the young cyclist. It is becoming very difficult for children to take their own places in a car-oriented environment.

Halloween evenings have been shown to be especially devastating: according to the CDC, pedestrian deaths increase fourfold among children on Halloween compared with all other evenings, despite the fact that Halloween is supposedly a children's day.[34]

Traffic accidents involving children are more frequent in poor neighborhoods[35-37] and on one-way streets.[38] There is a peak for injuries between six and ten years of age.[39] Studies of child pedestrian injuries from traffic carried out in New York and California showed that younger children were more likely to be hit at a midblock location close to home, while adolescents were more likely to be struck at intersections and at night; intersection accidents tended to occur further from the child's home.[40,41]

Toddlers are also at risk, but more often in the residential driveway when a vehicle backs up,[42,43] especially when there is no physical separation between the driveway and the children's play area.[44] The driver is usually a parent or a relative, and the vehicle is most often a truck or a sport-utility vehicle.[45,46]

Another automobile hazard for children, although less frequent, is becoming trapped in a car trunk. In July and August 1998, at least eleven children died from hyperthermia and asphyxia in such incidents.[47]

Often, children are blamed for being involved in traffic accidents, as if they were responsible for inappropriate street design, high-speed traffic, and so on, leading to child-oriented prevention strategies, which have been found to be less effective than environmentally based prevention strategies.[48,49] According to the Australian expert who studied this situation, blaming the victim serves to maintain the economic interests of the dominant groups in society, at the expense and suffering of children. Improving pedestrian safety is now mainly achieved by limiting pedestrian access to the street.

THE OLDER PEDESTRIAN

The elderly are overrepresented among pedestrian fatalities. As the streets become wider, the time needed to cross the street increases. But older pedestrians walk more slowly and take longer than younger ones to cross the street. A study carried out in six cities of the states of Washington and California found that even when crosswalk markings were present, the risk of being hit by a motor vehicle was still considerably high for older pedestrians.[50]

The National Institute on Aging in Washington, D.C., found that among 1,249 persons aged seventy-two or older in New Haven, Connecticut, less than 1 percent had a normal walking speed sufficient to cross the street in time at signalized intersections (i.e., four feet per second). Among those reporting difficulty crossing the street, 81 percent mentioned insufficient time to cross, 63 percent had difficulty with right-turning vehicles, and nearly one third had impaired vision.[51] The authors note that maintaining the ability to cross the street safely is fundamental to remaining independent in older age, especially in urban settings. Very often, the elderly cannot remain self-sufficient because their environment is designed only for those who can drive. In such cases, their admission to a retirement home may even be accelerated.

The safety of older pedestrians encompasses more than just their walking ability, however; they may also have difficulty judging the speed of oncoming vehicles, if they see them at all. Some elderly do not understand the meaning of international icons at crossing intersections, or are confused by the "Walk/Don't Walk" pedestrian signals, while others are unable to see them clearly.[52, 53]

The neighborhood environment itself was shown to have an impact on older pedestrian behavior, and on the health of the elderly as well. In an Alameda County, California, study, adults fifty-five years and older reporting multiple neighborhood problems such as heavy traffic, excessive noise, and poor lighting were at more than twice the risk of overall functional deterioration and more than three times the risk of lower-extremity functional loss one year later, compared with those who reported no problems in their neighborhoods, even after adjustments for individual demographic and health characteristics. Between 1994 and 1995, 6.1 percent of the cohort experienced incident loss of physical function, and 3.9 percent experienced loss of lower extremity function.[54]

The presence of walkable green spaces in the living environment of senior urban citizens was shown to increase the longevity of Tokyo inhabitants.[55] More than 3,000 older people were followed for five years, and their survival was found positively related to the quality of the physical environment near their residence—space for walking, tree-lined streets, less noise from automobiles and factories, and so forth—independent of their personal characteristics and health at the beginning of the study. The availability of such spaces near the home is believed to increase the opportunity of older people to walk outside and thus help maintain a good physical functional status in older age. This relationship held regardless of socioeconomic status, which is very interesting for the health and city planning debate. In Pennsylvania in 1999, older women who lived within walking distance of a park, walking trail, or stores were found to walk more, adding to the evidence of the environmental influence on physical activity. The ability to make utilitarian walking trips from home was associated with increased physical activity levels.[56]

Lack of physical activity has been linked to functional decline among elderly people. Those who reported walking at least one mile four to seven days per week were found to experience a lower level of disability of the lower limbs compared with those who did not report regular one-mile walks.[57]

TAXI MOMS

In 2002, the Surface Transportation Policy Project published the "High Mileage Moms Report" dealing with the burden of modern women living in suburbia.[58] According to this report, mothers are now spending more time in the car than ever before, taking care of family needs and driving the kids around—first to the daycare center, then to school, and after school to music or dance classes or to sports. The schedules of modern parents are regulated by the activities of their children, rather than the opposite, as was the case previously. The average mother spends more than an hour driving per day, traveling twenty-nine miles and taking more than five trips. Two-thirds of all trips for family needs are made by women, providing the transportation links that communities fail to offer to common destinations that cannot be reached by walking. Adding all these trips together make seventeen days in the car in a single year.

It has been suggested that many women spend more time driving than eating. They are paying the price of sprawl with their personal and family time, because driving limits the amount of time and energy they spend doing things with their families and erodes their quality of life. The way neighborhoods are now designed, with no facilities close to home, forces them to go farther for shopping and for personal needs. The absence of sidewalks also forces them to carry children around in order to protect them from the dangers of traffic.

Mothers drive to pick up and drop off their family members, mainly their children and older parents, as if they were bus drivers. They drive to the food store, the dry cleaner, the daycare center, the shopping center, the school, the park, and the playing field. Most of the time, there is no transportation alternative. Single mothers spend even more time in the car every day than married ones.

MOTOR-VEHICLE ACCIDENTS

Accidents are a problem not only for pedestrians. More than 40,000 people still die in motor-vehicle accidents every year in the United States, while 3.5 million are injured, despite improvements such as safer cars, greater seat belt use, stronger legislation against drunk driving, and better traffic signals.[59] The image presented by Hart and Spivak in their book about automobile dependence is a striking comparison: "During the 40 days of the Gulf War, the Americans lost 146 people on the battlefield, while in the same period of time, there were 4,900 fatalities on American roads and highways."[60] One in eighty-eight Americans will die in a car crash.[61] This is a frightening statistic. It might even seem unbelievable, but a simple calculation will illustrate this awful reality: since nearly 42,000 people die in car crashes every year, more than 3 million Americans will be killed in a car accident over an eighty-year period, which is now the average life span. As noted earlier, 1.2 million Americans died on the road over the twenty-five years from 1970 to 1995. Traffic fatalities have decreased during the last decades, but the decline has been much smaller in the United States than in Canada, the United Kingdom, or Australia.[62]

Imagine a small city disappearing every year from the country map. It seems like a science-fiction movie, but it is reality—the other side of the reality show, the side we would prefer not to belong to, the side of progress. We prefer to think of an accident as an act of God or as someone's fault, while in fact it should be attributed to excessive car usage, maybe not because there are too many cars, but surely too many car trips. The number of trucking accidents with fatalities reached 4,500 per year during the 1990s, killing 5,200 people.[63]

Here again, the fatality rate is higher in low-density cities such as Tampa, Atlanta, Houston, Dallas, or Phoenix, compared to higher-density cities such as New York, San Francisco, Portland, or Philadelphia.[64] A researcher from the School of Architecture at the University of Virginia at Charlottesville found that the central city and the inner suburbs bordering it had fewer traffic fatalities than the outer suburbs; these were the most dangerous urban areas, because cars move faster on two-lane roads, where driver impairment, mistakes, and inattention compound the dangers.[65] Comparing fatality rates and population density for fifty counties and cities in Virginia, the author of the study also found that denser places like Alexandria, Arlington, and Charlottesville had very low fatality rates, while less-compact cities showed higher rates.

Even at the county level, where you live is related to death on the road. In 448 metropolitan counties including nearly two thirds of the American population, a negative correlation was observed between traffic fatalities and sprawl: denser counties had a much lower fatality rate than counties with lower density. For every 1 percent increase in compactness, expressed by the "sprawl index" developed by the authors of the study, the traffic fatality rate decreased by 1.5 percent, revealing that sprawl is a significant risk factor for traffic fatalities.[66]

Young male adults are particularly at risk for traffic accidents. Car crashes are the leading cause of death among this age group. Many young men drop out of school to find a job in order to get a car as soon as possible. It is not surprising that owning a car has become the initiation rite marking the passage to the adult world. Without this magical instrument, the adolescent is entirely dependent on others for going places. Autonomy comes with driving, as it vanishes with the loss of the driver's license.

Beyond taking lives, motor-vehicle accidents incur annual costs of $230 billion, including $61 billion in lost workplace productivity.[67]

Other deaths are also due to motor-vehicle driving: more than 1 million animals are slaughtered every year on the roads, according to Defenders of Wildlife.[68] More wild animals are killed by vehicles than by any other means in the United States, compromising the survival of many species such as the grizzly bear, Florida panther, ocelot, Florida black bear, Canada lynx, Key deer, desert tortoise, San Joaquin kit fox, and Houston toad. The road network is also a threat to wildlife because it contributes to habitat fragmentation and degradation, as well as damage to water resources for many species, making them more vulnerable. Birds and other animals with large habitat requirements are particularly at risk.

AGGRESSIVE DRIVING

Driving usually occurs in a crowded environment, creating competition among drivers for limited asphalt space to get to their destinations in a specific length of time, the shorter the better. They also have to deal with people displaying all kinds of driving habits, often different from theirs. In this context, it is not surprising that drivers manifest some aggression—if not in their actual driving, then by intimidating or even threatening gestures. In the theory of sociobiology, "competition occurs when two or more individuals seek access to a resource that is somehow important to the fitness of each, and that is restricted in abundance such that optimal utilization of the resource by one individual requires that another settle for suboptimal utilization. Aggression is the proximate mechanism of contest competition. It takes place when individuals interact with each other such that one of them is induced to surrender access to some resource important to its fitness."[69]

Robert Park, an urban sociologist of the Chicago School at the beginning of the twentieth century—long before the birth of ecology and sociobiology—extended the competition hypothesis far beyond control for asphalt space. For him, "people compete for control of parks, streets, and ethnic districts—and above all for the prestige that comes from living in a fashionable neighborhood or having an impressive occupation."[70]

Because of the increasing amount of time we spend on the road and the growing number of car trips, aggressive driving has become a social problem that touches all categories of people; it is now becoming very common even among women.[71] This kind of behavior is encouraged by the anonymity inherent in car driving. Roads are more crowded than ever; everyone is in a hurry and gets very impatient when someone else is in the way, driving too slowly or changing lanes without signaling. The increase in traffic congestion and the resulting slowdown of circulation aggravates the problem; it lowers the threshold for exhibiting aggressive behavior. The street is a competitive world, and everyone on it competes for road space. This competitive situation explains why some people who are otherwise very nice, polite, and respectful of civic order become very aggressive behind the wheel.

Aggressive drivers have been estimated to account for two thirds of the deaths on U.S. highways.[72] Even though most of the incidents do not lead to criminal charges, the situation is nevertheless alarming. The aggressive behavior induced by competition on the road is rarely seen between two pedestrians because they are rarely in a competitive situation, and they cannot flee so easily. Even in high-density pedestrian traffic, where there is almost no room between walkers, the general rule is cooperation rather than competition; they trust each other and cooperate to avoid collisions.[73] According to Barbara Phillips, a specialist in urban life, unspoken rules govern pedestrian behavior, and these shared social understandings are the basis of public order.

Aggressive driving seems to be directly related to sprawl: the metropolitan areas with more aggressive-driving deaths are all recently designed suburban cities characterized by few pedestrian facilities and weak transit systems, such as Riverside-San Bernardino, Tampa-St. Petersburg, Phoenix, Orlando, and Miami.[74] In contrast, most metropolitan areas with fewer aggressive driving deaths are older, and their neighborhoods are characterized by the presence of grid street patterns, sidewalks, and more developed transit systems. Their residents can rely on other modes of transportation than car driving for their trips.

COMMUTING STRESS

Americans spent an average of nearly twenty-six minutes twice a day commuting to and from work in 2000, up from twenty-two minutes in 1990, according to the 2000 Census;[75] three quarters of commuters drive alone, putting a lot of pressure on the level of traffic and contributing to road congestion. The "High Mileage Moms Report," published by the Surface Transportation Policy Project in 2002, stated that the average American driver spent forty-three more hours per year in the car in 1995 than in 1990. In 1995, the average American spent 443 hours behind the wheel of a car, or fifty-five eight-hour workdays.[76] Sprawl has increased both the distance and the time it takes to get to work. The dream of the individual house in the suburb has given way to the nightmare of traffic congestion for those who live there. How many people decided to buy a house in the suburbs after a visit on the weekend, when the distance to work seemed shorter because there was no traffic, and realized after they moved in that the time spent commuting was much longer?

Traffic has become a source of stress, and commuting adds to the fatigue of the working day. *Time* magazine reported that the average American driver will spend six months of his or her life waiting for red lights to turn green, and over five years stuck in traffic.

Commuting stress has been shown to have physical and psychological consequences as well.[77] It is becoming difficult to plan arrival times, either at home or at work, because of the unpredictability of traffic congestion; one day it may take thirty minutes to get from here to there, while the next day it may take an hour, creating a feeling of loss of control. More parents come home too exhausted to cook or to interact with their children. Moreover, employees facing everyday traffic congestion are less productive and more likely to change jobs.[78]

The Annual Urban Mobility Report of the Texas Transportation Institute provides information about traffic congestion nationwide. In the seventy-five urban areas studied, the average annual delay for every person climbed from seven hours in 1982 to twenty-six hours in 2001. For these areas, congestion costs reached $69.5 billion, representing 3.5 billion hours of delay and 5.7 billion gallons of excess fuel consumed, averaging a per capita cost of $520 each year.[79] According to this report, the five areas showing the highest congestion levels were Los Angeles, Washington, D.C., Miami, Chicago, and San Francisco-Oakland. In many of them, rush-hour travel took about 50 percent more time than non–rush hour trips.

Unfortunately, the time spent in the car is not the only time devoted to the car. As long as thirty years ago, the average American already devoted more than 1,500 hours per year to it—both sitting in the car and working to pay for it, as well as for gas, tires, tolls, insurances, tickets, and taxes. All included, it totaled four hours per day; 80 percent of the time spent on the road was due to trips between home, work, and the food store.[80] Maybe the freedom theory should be revisited.

NEGLECTING TRANSIT

A smaller portion of commuters used public transit to get to work in 2000 than ten years previously, according to the 2000 Census Journey-to-Work figures: between 1990 and 2000, the proportion went from 5.3 percent to 4.7 percent.[81] In more than half the states, less than 2 percent of people were still using transit in 2000.[82] In the meantime, housing growth has been concentrated in suburban areas that tend to have poor transit service. More people drive to work because there is no other option where they live and work. Not only there are no commodities within a walking distance from home, but there is no transit either. A walk from home to the train station or bus stop would help people reach a higher level of physical activity. A majority of people said they did not use public transit because it was unavailable for the destinations or times they were traveling.[83] In fact, only 4 percent of the nation's 4 million miles of roads are served by transit. Nationwide, less than 2 percent of trips are now made via public transport; New York, however, stands apart, with public transportation accounting for a quarter of daily trips.[84] Cities where a higher percentage of people use public transit to get to work are characterized by a more compact and mixed-use type of development; they also have more residents walking to work.[85]

There is more than one reason for such a low level of transit use. First, many transit systems were driven into bankruptcy by automobile companies aiming to eliminate competition so they could sell more cars—and make more money. Second, the low-density development characterizing sprawl does not allow the development or survival of an efficient public transportation system; there are simply not enough residents per square mile to make it a viable option. Low-density development also means longer traveling distances. The viability of transit is linked to a high-density model of development. By allowing sprawl, municipal authorities have contributed to the failure of public transit. Finally, our car culture has put emphasis on subsidies for private transportation infrastructures, such as highways, wider roads, and parking facilities, at the expense of public transit investments. During the '90s, the federal government spent nearly four times more money for building and repairing highways than on mass transit.[86] We usually do not think much about the hidden costs of driving, but let's just mention that parking subsidies are estimated at $36 billion each year in the United States.[87]

The problem is not only with transit between the suburbs and the center of the city. Intercity transit is so inefficient and inconvenient in many parts of the country that only people without cars are using it. Once I took the bus from Fort Lauderdale to the Everglades in Florida—or I should say I tried to, because the attempt was unsuccessful. As mentioned earlier, I wanted to explore sites in Florida on foot, using mass transit to get from place to place. There was no direct bus to my destination, and I had to wait hours for a transfer. I finally reached a no-man's-land where the few residents working in a restaurant convinced me to go back where I came from, because it was too dangerous to stay around the area without a car. On top of that, the bus driver seemed to consider his passengers second-class citizens. Finally, it was a much more miserable and exhausting experience than traveling alone—even for a woman—through Turkey by night on a bus, as I had done a few years before the incident. It wasn't so much that Turkey is a safer country (although I believe it is), but that its extensive bus system provided a more secure and high-quality environment to its users.

Nevertheless, public transit expanded rapidly in the United States between 1995 and 2000, and in 2000 was at its highest level since 1959; the New York area accounted for half the growth.[88] The biggest increase was in rail transit rather than bus, partly due to the huge investment in new and expanded rail systems over the past two decades. But the fact is that a big part of our rail system is still underutilized, if not abandoned. Not far from my home, there is a railroad used twice a day by a freight train. The railroad goes from the suburbs to the center of Quebec, about five miles away. Since it is not very busy, it would make an excellent route for a light passenger train to transport suburbanites to the city, instead of congesting the 300-year-old center with cars. Visitors would be relieved of the nightmare of finding a parking place in the surrounding narrow streets, while residents could more easily find places for their own cars, as well as breathing cleaner air. But this model of development has not yet been favored, even though the benefits are obvious.

8

The Decline in Walking

Walking would teach people the quality
that youngsters find so hard to learn—patience.
—*Edward Payson Weston*

There are fewer and fewer places where people can walk, and also less time to do so. As a consequence, our perception of space and time has changed so much that the distance we are willing to cover on foot is shrinking all the time. The decline in walking is closely linked to the decrease of space in which to walk, and to the increasingly cruel lack of time we face—or think we face. Remember the last time you walked five miles in a row, somewhere other than in a park or in the woods while you were on vacation? Most people never do this; such a long walk just seems a pure waste of time and an exhausting experience. Why walk for so long when we could reach the destination much faster by car?

But the purpose of walking is not only to get to the destination. It is also a way to exercise and to get in touch with the physical and social environments. If getting to the destination faster is the main goal, how come we have less free time than ever before? Car driving speeds up the pace of life, but, strangely, it does not increase the amount of time available to do other things. It makes us simultaneously more restless and more tired. Walking less has even modified our physical appearance: people's bodies are becoming pear-shaped, and their muscles are wasting away.

Although walking is the most common leisure-time physical activity among American adults, it has been subject to a continuous decline. Data from the 1998 Behavioral Risk Factor Surveillance System indicated that only 38.6 percent of adults walked for physical activity, and among them, less than 40 percent met minimum current physical-activity recommendations (at least 150 minutes of walking per week, regardless of frequency).[1]

The number of trips made on foot has dropped by 42 percent in the last twenty years, even though more than one quarter of all trips made each day in the United States are short enough to be made on foot—that is, one mile or less (totaling at least 123 million car trips). Now, 9 percent of trips are on foot, and only 1 percent on bicycle. Much of the decline can be attributed to neighborhoods designed so that it is not safe or convenient to travel on foot.[2] Most of these areas were developed after 1950. They are mainly characterized by very low-density housing, the excessive use of curvilinear dead-end streets, wider streets, the absence of sidewalks, and no destination accessible on foot. Even a walk around the block has lost its meaning in an environment where dead-end streets prevail. Walking on some dead-end streets seems like invading someone's privacy.

The proportion of Americans walking to work is rapidly decreasing. Trips made on foot declined by 26 percent between 1990 and 2000, according to the *2002 Mean Streets Report*.[3] In 1990, nearly 4.5 million Americans walked to work, whereas in 2000, only 3.8 million did so. The degree of sprawl was found to be the most powerful predictor of walking to work in a study carried out for Smart Growth America; the proportion of commuters walking to work was one-third higher in more compact areas, compared with the least compact ones.[4] In Charlotte, North Carolina, fewer people walk to work than in any other metropolitan area of more than one million people; the city was also cited among the ten fattest cities in America.[5] Detroit, Dallas, and Houston are also at the bottom of the list when it comes to walking to work, with less than 2 percent of their residents doing so; at the other end of the spectrum, in the more compact metropolitan areas of New York, San Francisco, and Boston, more than 5 percent of residents go to work on foot.[6] Nevertheless, Canadian cities such as Montreal, Ottawa, and Vancouver scored better.

NEIGHBORHOOD CHARACTERISTICS AND WALKING

For lots of people, especially those living in the recent suburbs, there are no walkable destinations; they live too far from everything. For many others, going out for a walk seems hazardous because of unfriendly surroundings where crime, heavy traffic, noise, or dull scenery prevail. The only option left for walking is as a recreational activity away from residential neighborhoods.

Probably because until recently almost nobody paid attention to walking as a valuable physical activity, the understanding of environmental influences on this behavior is still limited. Australian researchers who reviewed the studies dealing with the subject in 2004 found that attributes associated with walking for exercise were different from those linked to utilitarian walking.[7]

Curvilinear streets not only increase the distance between two points, but are part of a hierarchical street design providing few alternative routes for drivers as well as for pedestrians and bikers; consequently they are also a risk factor for traffic congestion. According to Andres Duany and his colleagues, "Placing excessive curves and cul-de-sacs [dead-end streets] on flat land makes about as much sense as driving off-road vehicles around the city. . . . But there is a more serious problem: unrelenting curves create an environment that is utterly disorienting."[8]

Safety is also an important issue. The CDC analyzed data from the 1996 Behavioral Risk Factor Surveillance System in Maryland, Montana, Ohio, Pennsylvania, and Virginia, and found that people who perceived their neighborhood to be unsafe were more likely to be physically inactive. For older adults, physical activity rates were more than twice as high among those perceiving their neighborhood to be safe.[9]

An association has been found between age of residence and walking behavior in American adults. Those living in homes built before 1946, and from 1946 to 1973, are more likely to walk (one mile or more, at least twenty times a month) than those who live in homes built after 1973, suggesting an environmental influence on walking behavior. On the other hand, there was no relationship between age of residence and leisure-time activities such as jogging and running. The association between age of residence and walking behavior was present in urban and suburban counties, but not in rural ones. In older neighborhoods, destinations were not out of reach on foot, as they are in newer developments, because of more compact land use.[10] Surveys reported by the National Bicycling and Walking Study (1992) mentioned that walking on errands was important for respondents who walked, and distance was the main reason given for not walking more often. But when behavior—rather than motives—of people in sixteen U.S. cities was examined, density seemed a better predictor of walking than distance: the rate of walking appeared to rise as density increased.[11] This is probably due to the fact that greater density is associated with a higher concentration of services or other destinations, and therefore there are more reasons to explore the environment on foot.

Neighborhood characteristics such as sidewalks, enjoyable scenery, heavy foot traffic, and hills seem to encourage physical activity; when these characteristics are present, the neighborhood streets are the most common place for walking.[12] The streets have also been found to be the most frequently used facility for walking in Perth, Australia. Here again, access to attractive public open space, plenty of sidewalks in the neighborhood, and shops within walking distance are linked to walking for transport.[13,14] Despite the popularity of walking among Australian adults—72 percent of whom were found to have walked for transport, and 68.5 percent for recreation, in the previous two weeks—only a small proportion achieve the Australian recommended levels of 180 minutes or more per week; those who reach this level of walking activity have better access to attractive open spaces in their neighborhoods.[15] Australians reporting a less aesthetically pleasing environment are less likely to report walking for recreation or exercise. Walking companions—human or animal—were also important correlates of walking for exercise.[16]

The Missouri Cardiovascular Disease Survey carried out in 1999–2000 indicated that an environment lacking outdoor exercise facilities and perceived as unpleasant or unsafe—in terms of both traffic and crime—was associated with being overweight among adults; residents from such neighborhoods were one and a half times more likely to be overweight than adults from better neighborhoods, after adjustment for a variety of other factors. According to the authors of the study, population-level changes in health behaviors are unlikely to occur without the modification of underlying environmental factors.[17] In Australia, overweight was found to be associated with living on a highway or on streets with no sidewalks, or sidewalks on one side only, and with the lack of walking or cycling paths perceived to be within walking distance.[18]

The influence of environment on walking behavior was also observed in Canada. A set of neighborhood characteristics (including traffic threats, safety from crime, number and variety of destinations, social dynamics, walking routes, and others) was found to be associated with walking to work, whatever the degree of urbanization, supporting the utilization of traditional design concepts in urban development.[19] Density, diversity, and design can reduce motor-vehicle travel and increase walking and biking.

The *Transportation Demand Management Encyclopedia* from the Victoria Transport Policy Institute in British Columbia, Canada (available online at www.vtpi.org/tdm/index.php), has extensively reviewed how land-use patterns affect transport and has identified ways to improve land-use management and nonmotorized transportation. It was found that residents of mixed-use neighborhoods with connected street networks and traffic-calming devices such as speed humps, chokers, raised crosswalks, and roundabouts not only drive less than residents of conventional suburban neighborhoods, but are more likely to use alternative modes of transportation, such as transit, walking, and biking. The amount of land devoted to parking is also related to travel behavior; a large amount of parking space at a low price encourages driving over walking or public transit.[20]

DECREASE IN WALKING AMONG CHILDREN

In 1995, only 10 percent of children walked to school, compared to 50 percent in 1969.[21] Almost half of five-to-nine-year-olds now get to school by car. Children are less likely to walk to school in newer developments. Schools located at the outskirts of residential areas are increasingly isolated from the community they serve, leading to traffic jams when parents take their children to or from school.[22]

Yellow school buses have been part of the North American scenery for many decades. These days children are carried over longer distances to bigger schools that are far removed from home and often designed like storage buildings. At least, this mode of transportation is considered to be very safe: schoolbusinfo.org reported only twenty-five fatalities of pedestrians and eight of passengers in 2000. Overall, 5,500 school bus passengers and 500

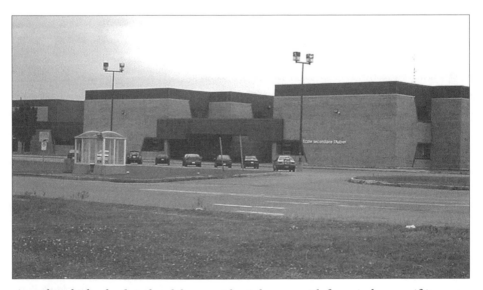

A modern high school, isolated from residential areas, with few windows, as if it were a warehouse. Children cannot easily walk to this type of school.

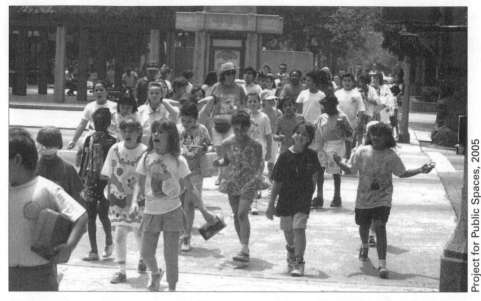

Project for Public Spaces, 2005

Children enjoy walking, but most of them are now deprived of such a simple and direct way to explore their external world.

school bus pedestrians are nonfatally injured each year.[23] Nevertheless, the fact remains that children traveling by bus do not have the opportunity to spend their surplus energy before entering their classes. The long trip can be tiring psychologically, if not physically. The sedentary way of life imposed very early in life on young children may have an impact on hyperactive behavior. A few decades ago, children had to walk about half a mile to go to school and would cross that distance four times a day if they returned home for lunch. Not so many were restless in class back then. Moreover, bus transportation is not free; its cost is over $400 per student annually, an expense not always taken into account when the location and size of new schools is being decided.[24]

According to the HealthStyles Survey of 1999, carried out among a representative sample of the American population, only 16 percent of respondents reported no barriers to their children walking or biking to school. Barriers included, in decreasing order, long distances, traffic danger, adverse weather conditions, crime danger, and opposing school policy. Among these reasons, traffic danger inhibited about 40 percent of children from walking or biking to school. Only 19 percent of children walked and 6 percent biked to school; the proportions were similar for primary and secondary school-aged children. Many children did not walk to school even when the distances were short. Among children who lived within a mile of school, only 31 percent of trips were made on foot. However, children with no barriers were six times more likely to walk or bike to school than those reporting one or more barriers.[25]

The perception of traffic danger leads parents to drive their children to school, aggravating the danger for those who do walk because there are more cars on the road. It seems that 20 to 25 percent of the morning traffic is due to parents driving their children to school, as reported by the Walkability Workshops held in June 2003 in Washington, D.C.

Data from the 2000 Georgia Asthma Survey indicated that in this state only, less than 19 percent of school-aged children who lived within a mile of school walked to school most days of the week in 2000, although walking to school provides a convenient opportunity for physical activity.[26] One of the national objectives for 2010 is to increase the proportion of children's walking trips to school to 50 percent for those who live less than one mile away. Georgia's rate of obesity more than doubled during 1991–2000, and it now ranks thirty-ninth in level of physical activity among school-aged children.

The decline in walking among children is now a worldwide problem. In the Australian cities of Melbourne, Perth, and Auckland, children's travel is characterized by high car use, low use of bicycles, and a steep decline in walking.[27] In Australian cities, even though the weather conditions are generally favorable for walking, over one third of children now spend less than five minutes walking per day. In Great Britain, the proportion of children walking to school on their own has decreased from 80 percent in 1971 to 9 percent in 1990, due in part to concern about the traffic danger, illustrating the barrier effect and the loss of a nonmotorized travel environment.[28]

Whatever the destination, children are less likely to walk than before: they now make 70 percent of their trips in the back seat of a car. The decline in pedestrian injuries among children has occurred at the expense of their mobility; fewer are injured because fewer are exposed to traffic as pedestrians. We restrict them for their own safety, increasing their dependence on adults willing to drive them where they want to go, and we force them to a sedentary life very early. By themselves, they cannot go to school, to the store, to the playground, or to visit friends. Often they are not even allowed to bike because it is too dangerous.

Because they do not have the opportunity to walk around by themselves, many children cannot explore their surroundings and learn to become independent. As they are not exposed to human diversity, their chance to understand those who do not share the same habits, values, or social

killed despite wearing a helmet. Most casualties are due to collisions with motor vehicles rather than to falls. Roads would be safer for bikers if there were fewer cars around, if traffic speed was reduced, and if more bike lanes were available.

Helmet wearing is a controversial issue and a very emotional subject. Studies trying to link helmet use with injury reduction are still inconclusive. Moreover, it was shown that other modes of transportation have higher head-injury rates as a result of road crashes. In Britain, for example, fatalities due to head injuries between 1987 and 1991 were 40.5 percent for car occupants, 39 percent for pedestrians, 12 percent for motorcyclists, and 8.5 percent for cyclists.[1]

It even seems that mandatory bicycle helmet laws—in Australia, for example—act as a deterrent to bicycling, thus canceling the health benefits of this protective device by decreasing the numbers of bikers on the roads.[2,3] Studies have shown that compulsory use of helmets reduced hospital admissions by 15 to 20 percent in Australia, but at the same time the level of cycling fell by 35 percent. Ten years later, cycling levels in western Australia are still 5 to 20 percent below the level they were before the introduction of the law.[4]

The emphasis on helmet wearing gives the impression that cycling is more dangerous than driving or walking, thus discouraging this mode of transportation. It has also led to neglecting the importance for bikers of following traffic laws as motor-vehicle drivers do, and to paying little attention to the promotion of a safer road environment. Wearing a helmet as a solution to the problem of biking safety is like using an oxygen mask to protect against traffic air-pollution: it does not solve the problem at its origin but constitutes only a patch to protect the victims—and maybe the insurance companies as well. Here again, the problem lies within the environment.

IS BICYCLING REALLY DANGEROUS?

In any case, biking is not as dangerous as people used to think. Many more pedestrians than bikers get killed every year. In 1996, there were 761 fatalities among bikers in the United States, one death for every seven pedestrians killed on the roads.[5] Compared to bikers, fifty times as many people are killed in cars or walking across the street, over forty times as many commit suicide, over thirty times as many are murdered, over fifteen times as many die from falling, over nine times as many are poisoned, over six times as many die of burns, and over five times as many drown, according to the

1992 statistics of the CDC. Whereas more than 90 percent of all cycling deaths are due to collisions with motor vehicles, the same proportion of all injuries is due to other causes that are less serious.[6] In his 1996 report, "Pedalling Health," Ian Roberts noted that less than 0.5 percent of injuries to cyclists are critical, compared to almost 3 percent for pedestrians, and that bikers have generally less-severe injuries following road accidents than other road users.[7]

Yet bicycling is a healthy transportation mode; there is no resulting pollution, no use of nonrenewable resources, no need for asphalting huge parts of the country, no induced traffic congestion, and no road damage; the health benefits of biking are well known, and they largely outweigh the risk of injuries. Cycling for half an hour a day burns 120 to 150 calories, providing a valuable way of controlling weight gain. Although bikers can be victims of traffic accidents, these accidents rarely compromise the health of pedestrians or other bikers. Without so many motor vehicles around, it would be a very safe mode of transportation. Statistics show that the risk of injury requiring hospital treatment as a result of cycling is much lower than for playing football, squash, basketball, or soccer.[8] Moreover, bikers are not subject to joint injuries, as are joggers. And the more cyclists there are on the roads, the safer cycling in traffic becomes.[9,10] Cycling for transportation rather than just for leisure would also help clear the air and thus reduce the occurrence of

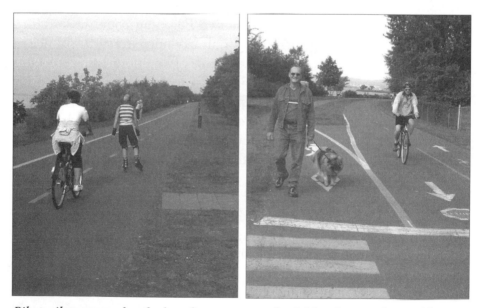

Bike trails are not only safe places for many types of activities; they can also provide a rare contact with nature for city dwellers.

respiratory problems linked to traffic air-pollution. Bicycling for utilitarian purposes would reduce traffic congestion as well, because there would be fewer cars on the road. Considering the fact that nearly half the trips made each day are three miles or less, bicycling could free up not only the roads but also seven-eighths of the parking space for an automobile.[11]

LESSONS FROM OTHER COUNTRIES

In a study carried out by researchers at Rutgers University in New Jersey, walking and cycling in the United States were compared with these activities in two European countries where they are a lot more prevalent.[12] In Germany and the Netherlands, where at least one third and nearly half, respectively, of trips in urban areas were made on foot or by bicycle in 1995, pedestrians and bikers were less likely to be killed or injured, both on a per-trip and per-kilometer basis. These two countries have drastically cut pedestrian and biking fatalities over the last twenty-five years by implementing a wide range of policies to improve safety, and by emphasizing people-oriented urban development. Between 1975 and 2001, cyclist fatalities declined by 64 percent in Germany—although there was a boom in cycling—and 57 percent in the Netherlands.

In contrast, the smaller decline in cyclist fatalities in the United States has occurred because of a sharp decrease in exposure to both walking and cycling. The policies adopted by these two European countries included better facilities for walking and cycling, traffic calming in residential neighborhoods, urban design sensitive to the needs of nonmotorists, restrictions on motor-vehicle use in cities, rigorous traffic education of both motorists and nonmotorists, and strict enforcement of traffic regulations protecting pedestrians and bikers. The city of York, in Britain, has one of the largest pedestrian and cyclist networks in Europe; prioritizing healthy modes of transport and restraining motor traffic has led to casualty reductions well above the national average.[13]

It was also found that Dutch and Germans who are seventy-five years of age and older make almost half their trips by foot or bike, compared with only 6 percent of Americans aged sixty-five and older. The elderly citizens of these countries get valuable physical exercise and also keep a level of mobility and independence that enhances their quality of life.[14] In the United States, bicycling is still concentrated among children and young men. Cycling sixty miles a week from the age of thirty-five could even add two years to life expectancy.[15]

I rent a bike every time I go to Europe—in France, Germany, Belgium, the Netherlands, Greece. As walking and biking are much more prevalent in European countries, one feels safer performing these activities over there. Cities are denser, making utilitarian biking more likely because there are more destinations at a cycling distance. I also used to bike in Cuba, where it is very safe because there is not much traffic. It seems one of the best ways to visit a country. While a rather long distance can be covered in one day, the speed is still on a human scale, so one can feel intermingled with the environment, smell the odors of the country, stop and interact with people, take a rest whenever necessary, and never get stuck in traffic. I never felt in danger biking in these countries because it is part of the culture, and so many people are biking that drivers have no other choice than to take care. At home, however, I often feel threatened by motorized traffic, especially in the city.

THE PLACE OF UTILITARIAN BICYCLING

Nearly half the trips made by Americans are three miles or less, and the use of a bicycle for these trips would simultaneously reduce traffic, air pollution, and the need for parking space; it would also bring mobility to the bikers, with all the known health benefits. The price of a bike rack is around $2.50, while a parking lot costs $20,000 per space to build.[16] It may take

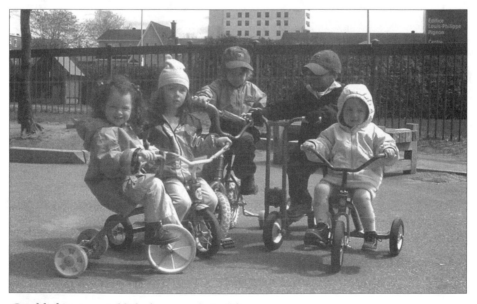

Good habits are established very early in life.

longer to reach one's destination by bike, but what do we really do with the time saved by driving? Is driving really time saving? It may be just an opportunity for more agitation. Driving is theoretically faster, but biking could potentially save time because of the resulting lower road congestion. Also, biking is affordable to almost everyone; and it can be performed by children and the elderly, contributing to their greater autonomy.

Although as many bicycles are sold as motor vehicles every year in the United States, bicycling has not yet taken its share of the road. Nevertheless, this fact reflects the increasing popularity of bicycling and the willingness to engage in such activity. But many people do not dare bike for transportation because of the risk of getting hurt by a vehicle; biking is for them only a recreational activity carried out on bike trails while on vacation. Dress requirements may also prevent some people from commuting to work by bike.

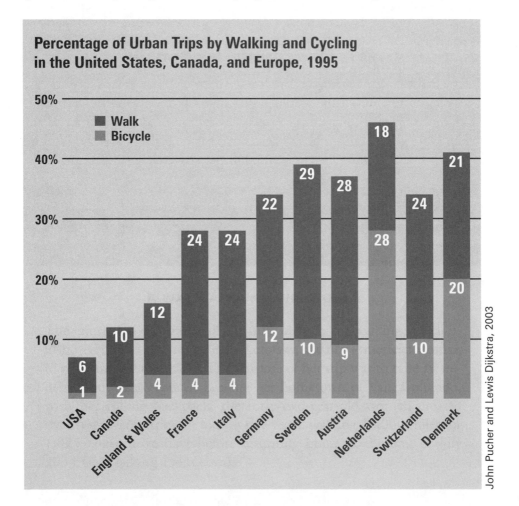

Percentage of Urban Trips by Walking and Cycling in the United States, Canada, and Europe, 1995

Legend: ■ Walk ■ Bicycle

Country	Walk	Bicycle
USA	6	1
Canada	10	2
England & Wales	12	4
France	24	4
Italy	24	4
Germany	22	12
Sweden	29	10
Austria	28	9
Netherlands	18	28
Switzerland	24	10
Denmark	21	20

John Pucher and Lewis Dijkstra, 2003

The percentage of trips made by bicycling in urban areas of the United States was only 6 percent in 1995, according to John Pucher, a transportation expert at Rutgers University who has extensively studied cycling trends in many countries around the world,[17] although there was a 55 percent increase in bike trips between 1990 and 1995.[18] Pucher reported that half of bike trips were social or recreational trips; utilitarian trips—including those for shopping, school, and personal business—accounted for less than half of cycling. As he mentions, in the most cycling-oriented European countries, two thirds of biking trips are for utilitarian purposes and only one third recreational. With a few case studies, the researcher and his colleagues show how the situation has improved over the past decade: New York, San Francisco, Seattle, and Boston are major cities where cycling has increased considerably. Among smaller cities, they examined the cases of Madison, Wisconsin, and Davis, California. To these they added Toronto, which was named as the best cycling city in North America by *Bicycling* magazine. These cities are very different in size, density, topography, and weather conditions, suggesting that utilitarian biking can be implemented in a variety of environments.

Utilitarian biking is more common in cities with a high proportion of university students and where the commuting distances are relatively short. University towns were found to have ten times the rate of commuter cycling that medium-sized cities do, which in turn have about one-and-one-half as many commuter cyclists as large cities, according to the *National Bicycling and Walking Study* published by the U.S. Department of Transportation, Federal Highway Administration, in 1992. This study stressed the complexity of the situation. No single factor explains a higher cycling rate. Cities with high levels (over 5 percent) of commuter bicycling usually have a population of fewer than 250,000, but smaller population size is not always correlated with a higher level of cycling. It was also found that in cities with very few or no bike lanes, there is not much interest in bicycle commuting. However, separate bike paths do not inspire bicycle commuting either; although they represent safe facilities for bicyclists, they are used more for recreational than for utilitarian biking. The authors suggest that this is because bike paths usually follow scenic corridors that do not necessarily lead to any major destinations. According to this study, a large number of bike paths is also an indication that bicycling has not been incorporated into the transportation network and is limited to its recreational function.[19]

Although utilitarian biking is more common in cities than in suburbs—because destinations are closer—very big cities with high-volume traffic on arterials or major traffic jams are not appealing to cycling commuters. According to Pucher, no city of one million population or larger, in either Europe or North America, has bike use exceeding 10 percent of trips.[20] Moreover, low-density sprawling areas can act as a deterrent to cycling, since everything is out of reach.

There seems to be a significant latent demand for utilitarian bicycling. Many respondents to American and Canadian surveys mentioned that bicycling would be their preferred mode of travel if suitable facilities and conditions—such as dedicated bike lanes, secure storage, and changing facilities—were available.[21]

10
Destroying the Landscape

Vancouver killed the freeway because
they didn't want the freeways to kill their neighborhood.
—*Rick Cole*

PAVING AMERICA

Half of Americans now live in the suburbs. What was rural landscape not long ago has turned suburban. As Marshall McLuhan said some forty years ago: "The motorcar ended the countryside and substituted a new landscape in which the car was a sort of steeplechaser."[1] The car brought homogeneity and uniformity to the urban and rural landscape; this fact is well reflected by the succession of similar restaurants found along highways and by the indistinguishable borders between adjacent cities. From 30 to 50 percent of urban America is covered with asphalt. This proportion reaches two thirds in Los Angeles,[2] with eight parking spaces per vehicle: one at home, one at work, the others at supermarkets, retail stores, restaurants, or other business establishments throughout the city.[3] Put together, these eight parking spaces require at least 2,000 square feet of urban real estate, which helps illustrate the cost of parking. Most urban streets have one or two parking lanes, accounting for 20 to 30 percent of their width. Moreover, a study reported by Todd Litman, from the Victoria Transport Policy Institute in Victoria, Canada, estimated between 125 and 200 million nonresidential, off-street parking spaces in the United States in 1991. After reviewing many studies on the subject, Litman came to the conclusion that much more land is used for transportation facilities than for buildings or any other structures, and that road space requirements increase not only with vehicle size, but also with speed. He showed that walking-oriented cities devote less than 10 percent of their land to transportation, whereas car-oriented cities devote up to 30 percent to roads and another 20 percent to off-street parking, highlighting the tremendous land requirements of the latter.[4]

THREATENING THE ECOSYSTEM

According to the Surface Transportation Policy Project, the U.S. road network has already consumed 17,375 square miles of land, an area about the size of Maryland and Delaware combined; 1.5 million acres of arable land are lost every year to road construction and sprawl.[5] Paving new roads and parking lots was found to reduce the ground's natural filtering capacity, causing increased siltation, runoffs of pollutants from impervious surfaces, reduced water quality, and increased flooding risk.[6] Moreover, the Sierra Club reports that floods are more frequent, and loss of life and property are greatest, in counties that have lost the most wetlands to development, because these were acting as natural sponges, soaking up and storing rain and runoff. When roads are bulldozed and asphalted, water that would have been stopped or slowed is now free to flood.[7]

Large paved surfaces increase the temperature of urban areas, which can get very uncomfortable in summer. Extensive land development is also a threat to wildlife habitat. In Massachusetts alone, forty acres are lost to development every day. Nearly two thirds of this land is used for low-density, large-lot construction—one-half acre or more—according to the Massachusetts Audubon Society.[8] Despite the decline in average household size, the living space for single-family homes has increased considerably during the last thirty years, as well as the average lot size, compromising the viability of ecosystems. Statewide, the average living space for new single-family homes grew from 1,572 to 2,260 square feet between 1970 and 2001, a 44 percent increase, although the number of people per household decreased from 3.12 to 2.51 during the same period.

Not only does sprawl consume more land, it requires more roads, more street lighting, and more extensive water and sewer infrastructures, increasing the costs of this type of development as well as dependence on fossil fuels. On these large lots, lawns and pools consume a lot of water, which can put great pressure on scarce water supplies. All citizens pay for delivering new services in more sprawling areas, whether they benefit from them or not, and it can be very costly, as reflected by higher property-tax rates.

LOSING FARMLAND AND RURAL COMMUNITIES

In Los Angeles, the population grew 45 percent between 1970 and 1990, but the development land area grew 300 percent, threatening productive farmland and aggravating traffic congestion.[9] Texas lost more prime and unique farmland to sprawl than any other state, nearly a half-million acres from 1982 to 1992.[10] On the other side of the country, the same happened in the Chesapeake Basin: between 1950 and 1980, the amount of land used for residential and commercial purposes increased by 180 percent, while the population grew 50 percent.[11] More than 90,000 acres are consumed by sprawl each year in the Bay states, and four to five times more land is now used per person than forty years ago, according to the 1998 Sierra Club report *The Dark Side of the American Dream*.[12] The extensive pavement and other impervious surfaces required by developments in the area also threatens the water quality of the East Coast's most important estuary.[13] The city of Phoenix covers 600 square miles, an area larger than the state of Delaware.[14]

The American dream, an individual oversize dwelling in a natural landscape, has begun to ruin rural landscapes as well, bringing traffic congestion to rural areas because the new residents still have to commute to work in the cities. Sacramento County, in California, is facing this situation, where "ranchettes"—parcels of land of around five acres—are devoted to residential development for people desiring a slower pace of life. Some concerns have already been expressed about endangering the ability to maintain a viable agriculture in these rural communities and the difficulty of serving these relatively isolated parcels with municipal services; state fire officials have attributed an increase in wildfires to the growing population in rural California.[15]

THE AESTHETICS OF SUPERSTORES

The new generation of stores—the superstores, also called big-box stores—have sprouted up all over the place. They are surrounded by a sea of asphalt that makes them uninviting for pedestrians. The asphalt is dangerous to cross on foot, and also risky for car collisions. These superstores are usually located close to highways and apart from residential areas, in such a way that they can only be reached by car. The whole environment has lost its pedestrian scale, and with it most of its natural beauty. Thousands of square

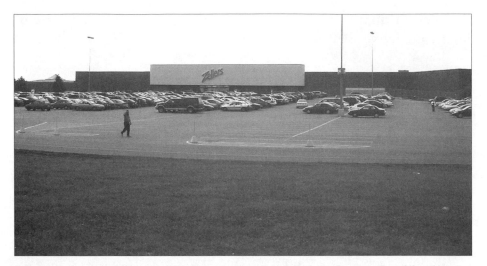

Stores where pedestrians could enjoy window shopping have been replaced by shopping malls that cannot be reached on foot.

feet on only one story, these buildings occupy a vast surface of land, and the huge space between the building and the street is devoted to car storage. Most of the time, their owners do not allow trees to grow in front of the building because it may hide their advertising signs. The pinnacle of ugliness has been reached by the multilevel parking garage, whether it is underground or over-; this waste of urban space is ugly from the inside as well as from the outside, and very often filthy and dangerous.

Although I am not a specialist, it seems obvious to me that huge low buildings cannot be anything other than ugly, because they are out of proportion. When it comes to aesthetics, the human eye is more attracted to height than to width. When we talk with pride about the size of a building, the height always comes first; the Empire State Building did not become so famous because of its width, but rather for its height at the time it was built. If a building is too low for its height, it is shocking to the eye, and it is difficult to find it beautiful. This type of commercial development is ugly in part because it does not take into account harmonious proportions in the design of the buildings. These considerations do not seem very important for those who build the structures, because they can be regarded as throwaway commodities, just like cars.[16] Low architectural standards have become the norm in suburbia, in contrast to the higher standards in the centers of old towns, where the presence of historic buildings inspires some respect for architecture.

Another ridiculous illustration of our cultural impotency is the drive-in restaurant, which combines ugly design and unhealthy food. By going there, you may save time, but often at the price of weight gain. How can eating in the car be an enjoyable experience? How can we have so little time that we are forced to eat in the car?

A lot may be more valuable as parking space than is the house built on it. Houses are often demolished to allow the construction of new roads, highways, and parking lots. People have to move farther into the hinterland. It seems that the car provides the opportunity to do so, but in fact there is no other choice. Asphalt and concrete have taken so much land—usually good agricultural land—for car use that people are pushed away to the end of the highway. And all there is to see on the way back home is a monotonous landscape covered with asphalt and lined with billboards and traffic signs, body shops, warehouses, fast-food restaurants, and motels. The highway strip is "a sequence of eyesores," wrote James Kunstler in *Home from Nowhere.* "This pattern of development is economically catastrophic, an environmental calamity, socially devastating and spiritually degrading."[17]

Urban riverfronts are often turned into freeways instead of public parks, depriving their residents of access to these precious natural sites. Roadways are infested with traffic signs and billboards that distract drivers, requiring a high level of concentration to process all the available information, especially at higher speeds, increasing the risk of accident. To be readable by those driving at high speeds, these signs must be oversized with bright colors and contrasts to catch the eye in just a fraction of a second, which necessarily makes the resulting landscape ugly from a pedestrian viewpoint. Property values along urban highways are always lower, and such properties are often the location of low-rent apartments. The aesthetic superiority of human-scale environments compared to car-oriented developments is not in question. The aesthetic degradation created by the latter bears a significant cost.

THE HOUSE AND ITS SURROUNDINGS

Reaching their destinations, commuters are greeted by a private, oversized home garage. Even house architecture has suffered from the car culture. Very often, the parts of a house that are seen first are the driveway and the prominent double garage door, rather than the porch of the house, which has shrunk over the years and is almost hidden, convincing strangers that they are not welcome. This picture has led to the expression *carchitecture.*[18] Houses seem to be built for cars more than for people. This kind of architecture provides few opportunities for informal social contacts with neighbors or strangers and creates an area inhospitable to the public realm, emphasizing the loss of community sense. Visiting such a neighborhood, a tourist from another planet could easily believe cars are the inhabitants of planet Earth: most of the time, they are the only moving objects outside, and they get into their garages by themselves before expelling their human content into the interior of the house, where the cars let their cargo feed themselves and sleep before sending them back to work the following day. This interstellar visitor would believe human beings are like slaves, working hard to feed cars and drive them where they want to go, and not the other way around.

The apparently harmless garage doors present a danger by themselves: every year, around 20,000 people are treated in hospital emergency rooms

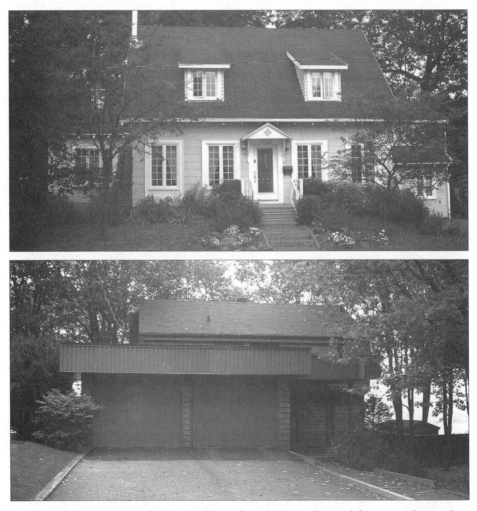

From architecture to carchitecture: the modern house is designed for cars. The porch as disappeared, along with the owners of the house. The front yard has become totally private.

for garage door–related injuries. Between 1982 and 1989, forty-three children were killed in automatic garage-door accidents, and many others were left suffering from brain damage or serious injuries.[19,20]

Where there are still sidewalks, they are built with a slope wherever there is a driveway, making it difficult for pedestrians, especially children and older people, to keep their equilibrium. The purpose of these slopes is to make smooth driving possible, but at the same time walking is compromised.

With the disappearance of sidewalks and the increase in traffic speed and density, the front yard and its connectivity with the neighborhood has been deserted for the back yard, strengthening the accentuation of private life at the expense of community life. The back yard is a private rest area where one can relax from the external agitation. Although it has become almost useless, the front yard is still very large, making the house look out of reach, and its occupants more or less like strangers to people passing by, decreasing its visual connectedness with other houses and the possibility of contacts with neighbors, leading to more isolation. The time when neighbors visited one another on front porches is over. The lawn surrounding the house reflects the monotonous homogeneity of the neighborhood and illustrates the impoverishment of the ground cover. So many beautiful wildflowers—now called weeds—have been eliminated to make room for this green outdoor carpet!

In her study of the public realm, Lyn Lofland observes, "Huge expanses of grass are said to be boring to children; city sidewalks, in contrast, are intellectually stimulating. Here they can learn how to relate to nonkin women and men, how to seek help when needed, how to move among crowds, how to take responsibility for people to whom one has no friendship or family ties, how to find adventure in mundane niches, and how to feel comfortable with different kinds of people, among many other lessons."[21]

Asphalt and lawn have become the two monocultures of urban America. No wonder cocooning has become so popular; it is so stressful and uninviting outside that it seems preferable to stay in, and look at the world through the television screen.

TRAFFIC CONGESTION

The generalization of car usage and the way our road network has been designed have led to lower residential densities, and this sprawl is usually characterized by segregated developments, housing being separated from business areas, stores, and schools, emphasizing even more the need for car transportation and aggravating traffic congestion. This extreme specialization of land use encouraged by zoning laws forces people to travel more, and the low-density pattern of development compromises the establishment or the existence of a good public transportation system. The absence of alternatives to car driving also increases traffic congestion. In his study of the costs of automobile dependence, Todd Litman, from the Victoria Transport Policy Institute in British Columbia, Canada, reported that automobile-dependent cities such as Los Angeles and Houston have much higher per-capita congestion delays than cities with more balanced transportation, such as New York and Chicago.[22] *The Miami Herald* reported that in 2000, over 42,500 miles of U.S. highways were suffering from congestion.[23]

Data from the Texas Transportation Institute on traffic congestion in sixty-eight U.S. metropolitan areas revealed that neither population growth nor too few roads were to blame for the rise in traffic jams. Instead, 69 percent of the increase in driving from 1983 to 1990 was due to factors influenced by sprawl—the spreading-out of development making everyone drive farther and more often to accomplish the same things.[24] It was also found that building new roads had little impact on congestion. In fact, the opposite is observed: increasing highway capacity causes more people to drive, until the equilibrium condition of crowding returns, according to Andres Duany and his collaborators. As these experts in New Urbanism have noted, "Trying to cure traffic congestion by adding more capacity is like trying to cure obesity by loosening your belt. Increased traffic capacity makes longer commutes less burdensome, and as a result, people are willing to live farther and farther from their workplace."[25]

A study carried out by the Berkeley Institute for Transportation Studies found that 90 percent of all new highway capacity added to California's metropolitan areas is filled within four years, and 60 to 70 percent of all new county-level highway capacity is filled within two years.[26] Widening highways and developing new ones induce more traffic by encouraging commuters to live further from work. Then, new road capacity leads to new traffic.

THE DESTRUCTION OF WALKING DISTANCES

The segregation of the different functions of the community brought about by sprawl has led to the destruction of walking distances and, with it, the destruction of walking as a normal means of human circulation, as observed by Lewis Mumford as early as 1961.[27] It is becoming more and more difficult to go somewhere on foot because destinations are not easily accessible.

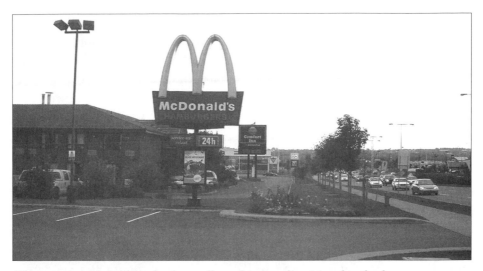

The same garish billboards along all roadways, advertising fast-food restaurants, gas stations, and motels, make it almost impossible to know where you are.

Too many people living in bedroom communities cannot buy milk or a newspaper without getting in the car. Although the shopping area may not be very far, roads are designed in such a way that it is impossible to reach destinations on foot. Curvilinear and dead-end streets increase the distance between two points compared with the traditional grid pattern. Because it is very difficult to know if one is going south or north, such streets are also disorienting. According to Mumford, we nevertheless nourish the illusion of the car taking us from door to door, even if we have to park at the edges of the huge parking lots surrounding shopping centers and workplaces. This segregation also adds uniformity and homogeneity to our urban landscape, resulting in a monotonous and unappealing environment for both residents and visitors. Sometimes it is almost impossible to guess where you are, because nothing distinguishes one suburb from another.[28]

THE EFFECTS OF ZONING LAWS

The main reason for zoning at the beginning of the twentieth century was to separate industries from residential areas, because the former were a major source of pollution. The industrial sector has changed significantly, however,. Antipollution systems have been implemented, and offices and stores have become the main workplaces. Having offices near your home is not harmful at all. But while the industrial situation of a century ago has changed, zoning laws have not; they are no longer appropriate for the type of economic development now prevalent. Most workplaces, such as high-tech industries, offices, and stores, contribute very little to ambient air pollution, but driving a car to get there contributes a great deal. Zoning laws dictate a model of development unfavorable to an aesthetic, healthy, and safe environment. James Kunstler, in his book *Home from Nowhere*, comments, "The model of the human habitat dictated by zoning is a formless, soul-less, centerless, demoralizing mess, producing suburban sprawl, and bankrupting families and townships." He suggests getting rid of these laws and replacing them with principles of civic art to improve the quality of the community.[29]

WALKABLE CITIES

If people really have chosen this kind of urban development, why don't they visit the suburbs while on vacation? Because the suburbs are dull, repetitive, and unaesthetic, and there is nothing to see or do there. Instead, people are going to older, more attractive—and denser—cities like Savannah, Charleston, Portsmouth, Boston, and San Francisco. But these cities' historic heritage is not their only attractive feature; they are also more pedestrian friendly, and because they were built before the automobile invasion, they are still on a human scale. The human scale is also what makes Vermont an attractive state, not just its beautiful landscape.

The destruction of walking distances struck me once on a trip to Washington, D.C., when I tried to reach my hotel from the subway station. I had made the reservation from home and had chosen the hotel because it was at a walking distance from the station. What I could not see then was that the road network was designed so I could not reach my destination on foot, even if the hotel was visible in the background. It was accessible to the eyes, but not to the feet. It was just impossible to go anywhere on foot without getting killed or at least injured. Highways and fences restrained human circulation, perhaps for our own protection. How strange is a world where pedestrians have to be protected from cars! Restraint is not the best way to implement protection.

Not very far from Washington are two much prettier towns: Annapolis, Maryland, and Alexandria, Virginia. Since these towns were built before widespread car usage, more emphasis was put on pedestrian travel. They are not only prettier, but also safer, which makes them more attractive and enjoyable for visitors as well as for residents. Many tourists visit these places because of their aesthetic and historic values, and because they were built on a human scale. Tourists rarely visit the suburbs. Such enclaves give me hope and make me believe it may not be too late to change the way things are now organized.

11

Street Democracy in Jeopardy

Any town that doesn't have
sidewalks doesn't love its children.
—*Margaret Mead*

THE DEPENDENT NONDRIVER

One third of the American population does not drive: the young, the elderly, the disabled, and the poor are left dependent on others for most of their trips. For them, the car culture has not brought any freedom at all: the urban design is adapted for car drivers only, and little effort is made to develop public transportation for other categories of people. These people face a loss of autonomy, especially when living in suburbia, where almost everything is out of reach on foot. In his book *Streets for People*, Bernard Rudovsky writes, "The American child presents the picture of a helpless baby, compared to his European counterparts; he cannot even make his way through the streets unaccompanied, and is completely dependent on others for going somewhere."[1]

Children now experience the world not directly, as they did before, but through technology—mainly television, the Internet, and video games. At the other end of the lifespan, the elderly have also become more dependent on others after giving up driving. A car-oriented type of development reduces not only the mobility but also the autonomy of a huge part of the population.

Car dependence leads to isolation for those who cannot drive, because cities are designed so that residential areas are separated from working places, shopping areas, and recreational sites. We easily forget that "we are all temporary drivers," as Jane Holtz Kay notes in her book *Asphalt Nation*.[2]

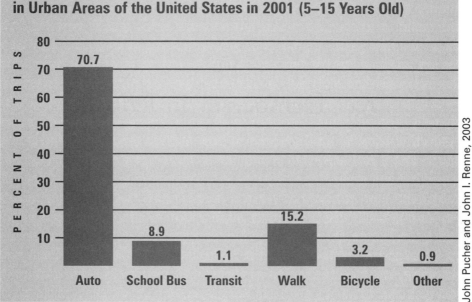

Children's Dependence on Others for Transportation in Urban Areas of the United States in 2001 (5–15 Years Old)

John Pucher and John I. Renne, 2003

We were all once too young to drive, and someday most of us will be too old to drive.

There are currently 19.8 million Americans older than seventy years who were still driving in 2003. As they get older, people are at risk of losing their ability to drive because of visual or sensorimotor impairment. They can then become dangerous on the road, like one elderly driver who killed ten pedestrians and injured fifty-seven others in July 2003 in an open market in Santa Monica, California, after mistaking the accelerator of his car for the brake. Once they lose their driver's licenses, older people experience a loss of autonomy, especially when there is no alternative to driving in their neighborhoods. This phenomenon will only increase as the baby boomers grow older.

The absence of alternatives to driving—public transportation, or walking and biking—may encourage some elderly people to postpone the decision to give up driving. It may also make it more difficult to withdraw driving licenses from motorists with poor safety records, which will increase the risk of accidents.[3] Losing the ability to drive has become the main step toward dependence in a car-oriented society; the resulting loss of autonomy is similar to losing the ability to walk, if not worse. First, no more car driving; then the wheelchair as a vehicle for those who did not walk enough to stay fit or were not lucky enough to remain healthy. Walking is such a normal activity that we don't realize its importance until we lose the ability to do so. The barriers to the disabled in wheelchairs are not exactly the same as those for pedestrians, but both groups experience similar frustrations and limitations in the course of daily life.

THE BURDEN OF DRIVING COSTS

A car-oriented environment is less equitable to the poor, because it increases geographical barriers to work and services; it jeopardizes their mobility by reducing the availability of travel alternatives; and it imposes a higher burden on low-income households for the purchase and operation of a motor vehicle. Because poor people drive less than wealthier people, they subsidize the well-off by assuming a disproportionate share of tax expenses for roads and parking facilities.[4]

The hidden costs of driving are paid by everyone, whether they drive or not. According to a special report, "Transportation Costs and the American Dream," from the Surface Transportation Policy Project, low-income families are disproportionately affected by car dependence: the poorest 20 percent of American households spend 40 percent of their income on transportation, straining their budgets and taking home ownership out of

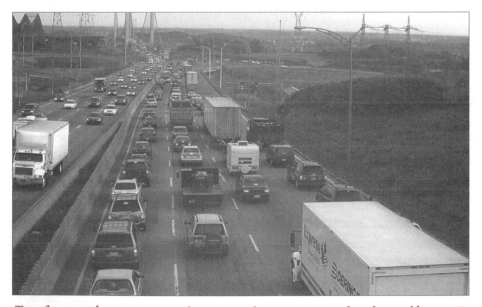

Too often, people must enter or leave a city by private car rather than public transit, bringing more congestion into the area.

reach because there is not enough money left to purchase a home.[5] Most American families spend more on driving than on health care, education, or food. For these families, the burden of transportation costs inhibits wealth creation. Very often, they own a car because where they live, there is no alternative to driving. This report also indicates that in more sprawling areas, families spend a much larger portion of their budget on transportation than in more compact, public transit-oriented or pedestrian-friendly areas; in Tampa, for example, the average household devoted nearly 25 percent of its expenditures to transportation in 2000–2001, while in New York, the proportion fell to 15 percent.[6]

STUCK IN TRAFFIC

To these victims of sprawl, we should also add the middle-class commuter, stuck in traffic congestion every working day. It has been shown that miles traveled increase as neighborhood density decreases.[7] An hour's drive to work twice a day is the equivalent of twelve weeks of work at the end of the year.[8] It is astonishing to see how the automobile has become a symbol of freedom, whereas in fact the health and financial burdens associated with its use are incredibly high.

ECONOMIC SEGREGATION

Sprawl—and zoning laws—have accentuated economic segregation in residential areas. A neighborhood of $500,000 homes will not allow the construction of houses half as expensive. Its residents will probably have similar earnings, similar cultural backgrounds, and similar values, which do not favor contact with a diversity of people and tolerance of social and cultural differences. Such people are also more likely to become NIMBYs (an acronym for "Not in my back yard," referring to the opposition to building public facilities in one's neighborhood).

12

The Vanishing of Social Cohesion

> The street, which is the public realm
> of America, is now a barrier to community life.
> —*Andres Duany*

THE DISAPPEARANCE OF THE PUBLIC REALM

More and more people now see the world primarily through the windshield, the television, and the computer screen, leading to more social isolation. Communal places where people of all ages, races, and beliefs can gather and socialize, even though they are strangers to one another, are disappearing. These places constitute the public realm, the social territory of the city. We now assist at the privatization of public space, a space not controlled by private individuals or organizations but open to the general public regardless of class, age, ethnicity, or other characteristics. Historically, public places such as urban squares and marketplaces played the role of arenas for public communication, where all kinds of people gathered and socialized. The public realm offers a rich environment for learning and operates as a center of communication.[1] In her book on the public realm, Lyn Lofland stresses the importance of the built environment as a medium of communication: "Space not only structures how communication will occur and who will communicate, it also has consequences for the content of that communication."

In Europe, sidewalk cafés also play this role; people feel at home and comfortable in the streets, because they can inhabit this public space instead of using it only for moving around. In the United States, the quasi–absence of sidewalk cafés and restaurants illustrates the fact that people have not appropriated the streets as part of their public life. It is probably one of the reasons why streets are more dangerous in America than in the Old World; their emptiness encourages misbehavior. On this side of the ocean, places like shopping malls cannot really play a social role, since their public space is owned by private companies that allow individuals to use it for private purposes only.[2]

AN ERODING SENSE OF COMMUNITY

The public space is narrowing while the private one is inflating, leading to greater segregation and atomization of society and decreasing the sense of belonging to a community. It is difficult to have a sense of community when you are working in one community, living in another one, and shopping and entertaining in a third, and when you can hardly distinguish one community from another. This aspect of the evolution of American society has been recently described with great acuity by Jane Holtz Kay in *Asphalt Nation*[3] and also by Duany, Plater-Ziberk, and Speck in *Suburban Nation*. As the latter note, "Community cannot form in the absence of communal space, without places for people to get together to talk. Just as it is difficult to imagine the concept of family independent of the home, it is near-impossible to imagine community independent of the town square or the local pub."[4]

This opinion is shared by many others, including Rebecca Solnit. "The democratic and liberatory possibilities of people gathered together in public," she writes, "don't exist in places where they don't have space in which to gather."[5]

As exposure to the diversity of the world lessens, public space is losing its educational possibilities for youth. The immediate environment has become too homogeneous to provide a variety of experiences; living areas are usually limited to people of the same socioeconomic strata. This homogeneity makes it difficult to distinguish one community from another in the suburbs. They all look the same and are surrounded by the same fast-food restaurants and strip malls. Lewis Mumford wrote of "an encapsulated life favoring silent conformity because it offers few opportunities for meeting, conversation, collective debate and common action." He also observed:

> Sprawling isolation has proved an effective method of keeping a population under control. With direct contact and face-to-face association inhibited as far as possible, all knowledge and direction can be monopolized by central agents and conveyed through guarded channels too costly to be utilized by small groups or private individuals.... Each member of Suburbia becomes imprisoned by the very separation

that he has prized: he is fed through a narrow opening: a telephone line, a radio band, a television circuit. This is not, it goes without saying, the result of a conscious conspiracy by a cunning minority: it is an organic by-product of an economy that sacrifices human development to mechanical processing.[1]

With the high degree of specialization of urban areas and the disappearance of walking as a means of circulation, the living tissue of the city disaggregates, and streets lose their social and political roles. As the words *city* and *citizen* have the same origin, it is not surprising to observe that civic life is now eroding because the collapse of the city itself has been accelerated since the onset of sprawl. Who can say where the center is of a sprawl city like Phoenix? Who can distinguish one city from another when sprawl obscures boundaries?

The sense of community can be maintained only when walking provides the opportunity for encounters of all kinds on a regular and informal basis. The million walking trips made by pedestrians in cities every day constitute the invisible threads at the root of civic life. Urban pedestrians spin the web of community and give true meaning to the word *citizenship*: participation in civic life. The solidity of the social tissue also depends on the existence of communal places such as squares, small parks, and cafés as mooring posts. Regular utilitarian walking provides opportunities for casual contacts with others and helps develop trust and commitment to the community. Relying almost exclusively on the automobile for transportation puts more emphasis on the private part of our lives because it decreases contacts among citizens, compromising the public component essential to the preservation of civic engagement. On the other hand, being surrounded with a lot of people, as in shopping centers, does not necessarily provide a sense of community. These places are filled with too many strangers with little chance to meet again to allow the development of any ties. They remain private places, even if walking is a prevalent activity there.

Contrary to common belief, the homogeneity of the suburban environment does not encourage social connectedness; rather, it leads to civic disengagement, as Robert Putnam shows in his book *Bowling Alone*. He attributes at least 10 percent of the decline in civic engagement and social capital to suburbanization.[7] The spatial fragmentation between home and workplace, and the increasing social and economic segregation associated with sprawl, disrupt community boundedness and lead to more isolation.

In Ireland, people living in highly mixed-use and walkable neighborhoods were found to have higher levels of "social capital" compared to the residents of car-oriented suburbs; they felt more connected to their community and were more likely to know their neighbors, to trust or have faith in other people, and to contact elected officials to express their concerns. They were also more likely to walk to work. The design of their neighborhoods enabled and even encouraged social ties or community connections. Their residents were more likely to interact in the course of daily life.[8]

Putnam showed how social capital and a healthy community are related: high-social-capital states have fewer violent crimes, their schools perform better, their residents are healthier and express greater support for equality and civil liberties, their kids watch less television, economic disparities are smaller, and so on.[9] It is not really surprising to see how a state built on a human scale, such as Vermont, performs well on this rating.

As James Kunstler has pointed out in his book *Home from Nowhere*, we now define ourselves as consumers rather than as citizens, as was the case fifty years ago. He writes: "Consumers, unlike citizens, have no implicit responsibilities, obligations, or duties to anything larger than their own needs and desires, certainly not to anything like the common good."[10] I suspect there may be a link between this new image of ourselves and the devastating epidemic of obesity. Consumers are in a passive state in which they accumulate things and act more like spectators. Even if they seem to be active, they ingest experiences as they ingest food, for their own good, without any consideration for other people. Consumers are by definition individualistic. As in the decadent Roman Empire, they feed on bread and circuses. In contrast, citizens willingly assume responsibilities and civic duties encompassing more than their individual needs and desires. They can be the initiators of revolutions or other kinds of political action. It is therefore not surprising that consumers are preferred to citizens by those who now make the rules.

GATED COMMUNITIES

The extreme social segregation (and social and economic homogeneity) is illustrated by the gated community; these residential areas with restricted access, guards, and surrounding fences where upper-middle-class people congregate constitute a rising phenomenon in the United States: more than three million American households are now situated in such enclaves, usually located in the suburbs, as shown by Blakely and Snyder in their book *Fortress America*. These communities appeared first in the Sun Belt states of the Southeast and Southwest, but they are now common in almost all metropolitan areas. Their emergence has political significance. According to Blakely and Snyder, the phenomenon "is a dramatic manifestation of a new fortress mentality growing in America. Gates, fences, and private security guards, like exclusionary land-use policies, development regulations, and an assortment of other planning tools, are means of control, used to restrict or limit access to residential, commercial, and public spaces."[11]

According to Putnam, these gated communities are innately introverted and represent a formalized and impersonal privatization of suburban life. For the sake of a safe and well-controlled environment, such communities adopt the principle of exclusion, in which empathy for others is not a natural issue.[12]

THE OCCURRENCE OF CRIME

Crime is more prevalent when the streets are empty, because there are no "eyes on the streets"—following the concept developed by Jane Jacobs in 1961—to witness the events that occur there and to create a sense of trust and solidarity among members of the community. It surely feels safer to walk on a street when all kinds of people are present than when you are alone. Jane Jacobs elucidated the role of a city's streets and sidewalks in keeping the city safe. According to her, a lively street not only has users, but also watchers. The kind of single-use environment characterizing sprawl means that many parts of a city are empty for an important part of the day: residential areas during the day when everyone is at work, workplaces and shopping areas at night. This single occupancy makes an area more vulnerable to deviant behavior because there is no surveillance and no social pressure to restrain it. *Eyes on the streets* not only means more pedestrians on the streets, it means more buildings with windows facing the street instead of plain walls. People watching from windows can act as a deterrent to crime or misconduct just by being there. The concept also means active street life generated by mixed-use neighborhoods, where the different functions of the city are intermingled—housing, working, shopping, and entertaining all found in the same area to provide an around-the-clock occupancy. The social cohesion created by this intermingling of the multiple functions of society has been shown to be inversely related to the prevalence of violent crime.[13] By increasing community cohesion, environmental design focused on walkability may help reduce crime and other social problems.

THE SOCIAL ROLE OF SIDEWALKS

Jane Jacobs has devoted many chapters of her book on the design of American cities to the social role of sidewalks. In addition to the opportunities for contacts between people, they offer educational possibilities for children. She points out that children are under closer adult supervision on the sidewalks than they are in recreational parks, and consequently safer. Supervision does not need to be done exclusively by parents but can be provided by neighbors, thus sharing the burden among adults.

When sidewalks are public places informally used by all kinds of people, they provide safe opportunities for contacts. This quality of safety relies mainly on trust:

> The trust of a city street is formed over time from many, many little public sidewalk contacts. It grows out of people stopping by at the bar for a beer, getting advice from the grocer and giving advice to the newsstand man, comparing opinions with other customers at the bakery and nodding hello to the two boys drinking pop on the stoop, eyeing the girls while waiting to be called for dinner, admonishing the children, hearing about a job from the hardware man and borrowing a dollar from the druggist, admiring the new babies and sympathizing over the way a coat faded.[14]

THE PRESENCE OF FAMILIAR STRANGERS

Relying on cars for transportation does not provide much social contact in the neighborhood. The absence of pedestrians jeopardizes the sense of solidarity existing between "familiar strangers": according to the concept developed by the American social psychologist Stanley Milgram in 1972, even if we do not personally know the people we meet on the street on a regular basis, they become part of our life, and a special link is created between us. They form a border zone between people we know and the complete strangers we encounter once and never see again.[15] This link is made of mutual trust and reveals itself mostly when a catastrophic or at least an unusual event occurs. It is the kind of link reported between New Yorkers on September 11, 2001. Suddenly, the usual individualism gave way to solidarity among people not related to each other but only juxtaposed in normal life. Familiar strangers are more prone to help each other in such a situation than in normal life.

I remember when my family moved after living twenty-five years in the same house in a small town. Some neighbors came to say goodbye to my mother, although it was the first time they had come to our house in a quarter of a century. They had raised their children side by side with us, but they had never interacted with our family. They were like strangers. Not exactly, however; they were *familiar* strangers, and I am sure that if something had happened to one of them, the others would have been there to help. They

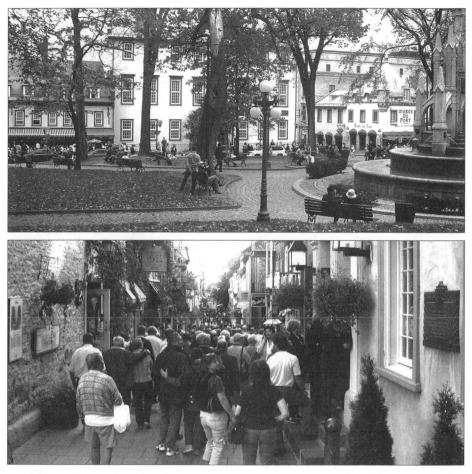

Streets and urban spaces can facilitate contacts between people and create opportunities for them to gather.

shared the same life situation, although they did not have any formal connection. This trend is disappearing with sprawl. Since most trips are made by car, neighbors rarely meet. They do not share the same social space, and they do not need to trust each other.

THE POLITICAL ROLE OF THE STREET

A powerful social cohesion among citizens also appears during political and antiwar demonstrations, and then one can easily understand why these events always involve pedestrians. It would never occur to anybody to protest against war by car. Marches to raise money for humanitarian causes proceed from the same elements.

Marches play an important role as part of the democratic process. They are organized to rouse public opinion on important issues and bring them into the forefront of political debate. This form of gathering speaks its own language; the movement of the crowd symbolizes the action toward a common goal. Such mass demonstrations can be very effective in influencing political decisions and bringing about social change. Over the past century, most political protests used the term *march* to describe these movements on civil rights, racial discrimination, peace, disarmament, or ecology. The term was borrowed from the French, renowned for centuries for their way of addressing political issues in the streets.

Public places where people can gather make humans equal and bind them together toward a common goal, whether it is a religious festival, carnival, or political activism, or any other kind of cultural expression. It is one of the best ways to express oneself as a citizen. In this regard, the renewal of pilgrimages highlights the importance given to such ties among human beings. With great insight, Rebecca Solnit has written, "When public spaces are eliminated, so ultimately is the public; the individual has ceased to be a citizen capable of experiencing and acting in common with fellow citizens. Citizenship is predicated on the sense of having something in common with strangers just as democracy is built upon trust in strangers. And public space is the space we share with strangers, the unsegregated zone."[16]

Walking and revolutions were tightly intermingled in history. The French Revolution more than 200 years ago, and more recently the Portuguese and Czech revolutions, involved public manifestations carried out by pedestrian citizens. Maybe that is why planners and political authorities have favored the creation of an environment incompatible with walking. When people are confined to the private sphere, it is more difficult for them to gather and share common values with strangers. It is more difficult for them to protest against the imposed rules. And they are easier to keep under control.

In contrast, the private car makes us competitors; it simultaneously isolates and marks the social status of its owner. Everybody wears jeans, but driving an Audi or a Lexus is not for everyone. The car is such a powerful ego-reinforcement that it would be unrealistic to try to convince people to abandon it.

Pedestrians sharing a public space are more equal, and this sense of equality between strangers is needed for a common action. When the opportunity to participate in events involving pedestrians shrinks, so does the citizen's role. Not being able to assume their social role as a group, people may also lose their power as individuals.

13

Traffic Air Pollution

There's so much pollution in the air now
that if it weren't for our lungs there'd be no place to put it all.
—*Robert Orben*

A STRANGE FEELING IN THE LUNGS

On a beautiful sunny August morning during a vacation trip to Manhattan Beach, just south of Los Angeles, I decided to go for a bike ride to Marina del Rey on the paved path along the sea, about a twelve-mile ride. I came back with an unusual pain in my chest. It was not the kind of pain you get when doing too much exercise—I was used to biking longer distances on more difficult roads—but the feeling of breathing contaminated air. Because I had been breathing deeply along the way, the level of ozone concentration in my lungs was probably higher than usual. Everyone knows that sometimes the level of smog is too high to allow outdoor exercise in the Los Angeles area. Even though there was no smog alert on this Sunday morning, I could feel the effect of air pollution inside my lungs, despite the proximity of the sea.

The problem recently inspired researchers in their choice of a title for a scientific article on the subject: "Breathless in Los Angeles: The Exhausting Search for Clean Air." The Children's Health Study, one of the largest surveys of the long-term consequences of air pollution on the respiratory health of children, was carried out in Southern California. Six thousand public school children from twelve different communities were followed for many years. It was found that lung development was approximately 10 percent slower among children living in communities with higher levels of nitrogen dioxide (NO_2, from car exhaust) and other traffic-related pollutants, including nitric acid vapor and particulate matter. An improvement was seen, however, among children who moved away from the polluted communities. School absence rates increased when ozone levels rose. Children with asthma experienced more bronchitis when living in communities with more NO_2 or particulate pollution. Children who played team sports and spent more time outside in communities with high ozone levels were found to have a higher incidence of newly diagnosed asthma.[1]

DRIVING AS A SOURCE OF AIR POLLUTION

Driving is one of the main sources of air pollution. The release of carbon monoxide, carbon dioxide, nitrogen oxides, hydrocarbons, and fine particulate matter has a deleterious effect on the respiratory system, leading to the death of over 64,000 Americans every year from illnesses caused by air pollution.[2] Moreover, nitrogen oxides and hydrocarbons together in the presence of sunlight form ozone, an airway irritant responsible for a higher incidence and severity of respiratory symptoms.[3] According to the Surface Transportation Policy Project, more than 125 million Americans live in areas with unacceptable air pollution; nearly 15 million of them suffer from asthma, and this disease causes over 1.5 million emergency department visits, about 500,000 hospitalizations, and over 5,500 deaths every year.[4] High ozone levels are associated with higher incidence and severity of respiratory symptoms, worse lung function, more emergency room visits and hospitalizations, more medication use, and more absenteeism from school and work.[5] Car driving is also one of the main sources of greenhouse gas emissions, contributing to the global warming of the planet and its consequences for the disappearance of species. These pollutants are not only present in the environment but also inside the car that is stuck in traffic, regardless of the type of vehicle and its ventilation settings;[6] driving in dense traffic can lead to interior concentrations of pollutants up to ten times higher than in ambient city air. The situation persists even when windows and vents are closed.

DIFFERENCES ACCORDING TO WHERE YOU LIVE

Since sprawl is associated with high levels of driving, more air pollution results from this kind of urban development, aggravating the occurrence of respiratory health problems. The degree of sprawl has been found to be strongly related to the severity of maximum ozone days.[7] It is not a coincidence that the most sprawling of U.S. metropolitan areas—Riverside–San Bernardino, California—also has the highest number of days of unhealthy air quality (445 days from 2000 to 2002).[8] According to Smart Growth America, 90 percent of total cancer risk in the Los Angeles Basin is attributable to toxic air pollutants emitted by mobile sources. The smog of Los Angeles degrades air quality even as far away as the Grand Canyon in Arizona, hundreds of miles distant.[9]

Clearing the Air, a report published by the Surface Transportation Policy Project in 2003, shows how much air pollution you are exposed to in your area of residence. It gives the air-quality index for more than fifty metropolitan areas nationwide and the air pollution trend over the last decade. It also estimates for each area the level of pollution from cars, buses, and trucks, and the public health costs resulting from air pollution. For Los Angeles alone, transportation-related public health-care costs from air pollution were estimated at $1.8 billion for the year 2001. Between 2000 and 2002, the five metropolitan areas with the highest number of days of unhealthy air quality were all located in southern California, although their ozone levels were on the decline. They included Riverside–San Bernardino, Fresno, Bakersfield, Los Angeles–Long Beach, and Sacramento; all had more than 150 days of unhealthy air quality during the three-year period 2000 to 2002.[10] Motorized transportation was found to be responsible for the release of about two thirds of the carbon monoxide in the atmosphere, one third of nitrogen oxide, 29 percent of hydrocarbon emissions, and 10 percent of fine particulate matter; all these increase cancer risk and heart-disease prevalence. Gains from vehicle technology improvements following the Clean Air Act of 1970 and the Congestion Mitigation and Air Quality Improvement Program of 1991 are offset by the huge increase in driving—more trips and more miles driven per trip—leading to heavy public health costs, between $40 billion and $64 billion per year, the greatest part attributable to premature death.

Both increases in household and employment density and better street connectivity decrease vehicle mileage, travel time, trips, and the need for cold starts, reducing air-pollution emissions because there are substitutes for driving, such as walking and public transit.[11] All these characteristics are absent from sprawling areas.

A MAJOR SOURCE OF RESPIRATORY PROBLEMS

The level of air pollution has been correlated with increased emergency visits for asthma in Cincinnati, Cleveland, and Columbus, Ohio;[12] in

Atlanta;[13] and in Seattle.[14] Air pollution levels were also found to be related to an increased risk of mortality in many other cities.[15–17] These problems are aggravated by the massive tree loss in American cities, due primarily to urban sprawl and highway construction. In the past ten years, 20 percent of trees have disappeared in urban areas, according to the environmental group American Forests, which considers this factor responsible for the rise in respiratory diseases. The study of 448 urban areas used satellite imagery to compare the tree cover with what had been observed ten years previously.[18] It is well known that trees remove pollution from the air; they also cool the environment and reduce the need for air conditioning, as reported by Reuters on the Environmental News Network.[19]

During the seventeen days of the 1996 Summer Olympic Games in Atlanta, the number of asthma acute-care events among children (hospitalizations and emergency-care visits) decreased substantially, following the city's effort to reduce traffic congestion via the development of a twenty-four-hour public transportation system and the closure of a downtown sector to private automobile travel, which reduced the levels of ozone, particulate matter, and carbon monoxide concentration in the air. The benefits were almost immediate and weigh strongly in favor of major changes in commuting behavior to improve the respiratory health of urban residents.[20]

The impact on health problems of high levels of traffic air-pollution in a neighborhood has been studied extensively in Europe. Positive associations were found in Germany between wheezing and allergic rhinitis among children and adolescents, and self-reports of traffic density on street of residence,[21,22] and between reduced pulmonary function, increased respiratory symptoms, and objective measures of traffic density.[23] Recurrent bronchitis, bronchiolitis, and pneumonia among children and adolescents were related to the intensity of truck traffic in northern Italy.[24] In the Netherlands, respiratory symptoms such as cough, wheeze, runny nose, and doctor-diagnosed asthma were found more commonly among children living within 300 feet of the highway, with greater exposure to truck traffic, compared with children living further away;[25] poorer lung function was also observed.[26] In the city of Birmingham, England, children hospitalized for asthma were more likely to live in an area with a high traffic flow.[27]

ALSO RESPONSIBLE FOR PREMATURITY

Unfortunately, traffic air pollution is not related only to respiratory problems: it was recently found that exposure during pregnancy can increase the risk of preterm birth and low birth weight. A study carried out in Los Angeles County involving nearly 51,000 infants born between 1994 and 1996 showed a 10 to 20 percent increase in the risks of preterm birth and low birth weight in infants born to women living close to heavily traveled roadways, even after controlling for socioeconomic status and other factors. The study took into account residential proximity to, and level of traffic on, roadways surrounding homes. These adverse outcomes occurred more often when the third trimester of pregnancy fell during the autumn or winter months, because more stagnant air conditions prevailed at this time of the year.[28]

SUMMING UP THE CONSEQUENCES

Considering all the adverse effects of how cities are now designed and the resulting importance given to car driving, it is quite surprising that so little attention has been paid until now to a global approach to the problem of walking less. One of the reasons might be that pedestrians, unlike other consumer or citizen groups, are still not very well organized to protect their own rights. Unless they are marching for a specific cause, they are rather isolated. But a window of opportunity seems to be opening now that urban planners, transportation experts, and public health specialists are beginning to work together. Many advocacy groups have emerged to promote greater safety on the road and healthier lifestyles; they are asking for increased funding for the creation of pedestrian-friendly environments. These organizations—among them Safe Routes to School, America Walks, Partnership for a Walkable America, and the League of American Bicyclists—are trying to improve walking and cycling conditions and to increase the number of people engaged in such activities.

Perhaps the obesity crisis will be a more convincing argument for developing walkable communities than are the huge numbers of people dying or being injured on the road every year, the time lost in traffic, the shrinking of the public realm, or the increase in respiratory problems due to air pollution. Since walking was at first and until very recently a utilitarian activity, restoring it as part of daily life could help people achieve the recommended levels of physical activity.

Part 3

The Burden
of a Sedentary Lifestyle

14

The Decline in Physical Activity

We are underexercised as a nation.
We look instead of play. We ride instead of walk. Our existence deprives
us of the minimum of physical activity essential for healthy living.
—*John F. Kennedy*

Although sports have taken an important place in our leisure time, we find ourselves most often watching the games on TV, rather than participating. Even when people attend a football game, they are sitting down watching a few others engage in strenuous physical activity. As spectators, we often ingest large amounts of fast food. Sedentary life encourages overeating, and overeating induces sedentary life. Yes, we like sports, but we tend to prefer watching to participating. Unfortunately, many people mistakenly assume that exercise can be provided only by sports, instead of by daily-life activities such as walking, gardening, lawn mowing, stair climbing, or leisure activities like bowling and dancing. Although these are not vigorous activities, they nevertheless allow beneficial energy expenditure when performed on a regular basis.

Physical inactivity as a consequence of our sedentary lifestyle has now become a serious public health issue. In 2002–2003, 25 percent of Americans over age eighteen reported having mobility limitations for walking, standing, or climbing stairs.[1] Physical inactivity is now considered responsible for 250,000 to 300,000 deaths caused by heart attack and stroke annually in the United States alone. In men, the risk of a heart attack from being sedentary is similar to smoking twenty cigarettes a day, having a systolic blood pressure over 150 mmHg, or having a blood cholesterol over 6.9 mmol/L.[2]

Even though a lot of people are concerned with physical fitness, the fact is that we spend more and more time sitting down—in the car or in front of the TV or the computer. As if that were not enough, the remote control accentuates this state of passiveness.

Most of us now have a sedentary job and get there by car; a few decades ago, the work situation required more physical activity, and more people walked to work. According to a British survey, only 20 percent of men and 10 percent of women were still employed in occupations requiring significant physical activity at the beginning of the '90s; moreover, one third of adults had undertaken fewer than four twenty-minute periods of any type of moderate activity in the previous month, and more than 80 percent did not walk continuously for at least two miles.[3] Free time has increased over the last decades, but most of the increment has gone to sedentary activities.

With the increasing pace of life, many people are always in a rush and do not even have enough time to cook. Despite sophisticated kitchens equipped with modern amenities, the proportion of dinners purchased from a takeout counter or a grocery freezer increased by 24 percent in the past decade.[4] Home-cooked meals are becoming less popular: according to the special report "Cut the Fat" published in the January 2004 edition of *Consumer Reports*, 46 percent of the total food budget was spent on meals away from home in 2002, compared to 37 percent in 1977.[5] Food eaten outside the home is generally higher in fat than food prepared at home. Moreover, cooking requires time and an upright posture, as does cleaning up the kitchen after the meal; eating from the throwaway container of a prepared meal is often much simpler. The kitchen is becoming an asset mainly for show: we may contemplate it from the living room, since it can often be seen from this open area, but its utility is vanishing. Like the fireplace, it seems to be a remnant from another era, more a decoration than a necessity.

Office work now means sitting in front of a computer for long hours in such a tiny space that you do not even have to stand up to get a file from the drawer. Saving space has become a key value for any company. For the office worker, it also means saving energy. There are not many opportunities for exercise on the work site. And trying to concentrate with the surrounding noise is often an exhausting experience. Repetitive strain injuries, such as carpal tunnel syndrome and epicondylitis, from computer use are common, and it can take a long time to recover from them.

A national survey carried out in 2000–2001 revealed that more than half of American adults did not meet the minimum recommendation for physical activity (at least thirty minutes a day for five days or more per week). At the national level, 26 percent were totally physically inactive in their leisure time; in some states (Kentucky, Louisiana, Mississippi, and Tennessee), one in three adults was totally physically inactive during leisure time.[6] The situation is similar for children. They now spend three quarters of their waking hours being inactive, engaging in vigorous physical activity for as little as twelve minutes per day.[7]

Some of us prefer not to engage in physical activity because we do not enjoy a strenuous, or at least a vigorous, workout in which we have to sweat a lot and suffer a bit. We do not hear much about the benefits of light or moderate activity. It now seems, however, that physical activity has a cumulative beneficial effect: it is not necessary to perform it for hours at a time; small amounts every day add up. It does not have to be a sport, either. Many people do not like sports, or do not have money for the equipment. Perceiving physical activity as limited to sports, they prefer to refrain. As a kid, I did not like the competitive side of sports, but being more nature-oriented, I was attracted by the adventurous side of hiking and biking.

A study involving 448 counties in the largest metropolitan areas nationwide between 1998 and 2000 revealed that residents from the twenty-five most sprawling counties walked an average of 191 minutes a month, compared with 254 minutes a month among those living in the twenty-five densest counties. The degree of sprawl was related not only to walking, but also to overweight and high blood pressure. Residents of the most spread-out areas weighed about six pounds more on average than those living in the most densely populated places.[8] Interestingly, people do not necessarily walk more where there is mild weather, since denser areas are more often located in the northern part of the country.

PHYSICAL INACTIVITY AND HEALTH

A sedentary lifestyle contributes to many diseases including obesity, diabetes, coronary heart disease, stroke, osteoporosis, some cancers, and all-cause mortality. According to the CDC, sedentary living is responsible for about one third of deaths due to coronary heart disease, colon cancer, and diabetes; just a small increase in physical activity would reduce mortality from these conditions by as much as 5 to 6 percent, or 30,000 to 35,000 deaths per year.[9]

Our sedentary lifestyle is echoed in the use of our leisure time. The absence of leisure-time physical activity has been found to be responsible for

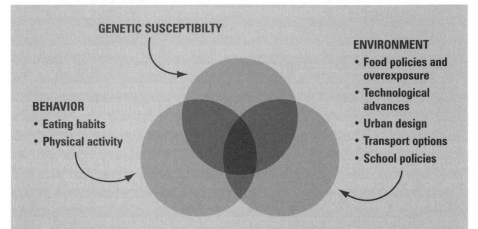

GENETIC SUSCEPTIBILTY

ENVIRONMENT
• Food policies and overexposure
• Technological advances
• Urban design
• Transport options
• School policies

BEHAVIOR
• Eating habits
• Physical activity

Interaction Between Personal and Societal Factors Leading to Obesity

While genes can make a person more prone to obesity, behavior and environment are really the determinants. Although our behavior is ultimately under our personal control, our behavioral choices now are made in an overwhelmingly obesogenic environment.

Food policies and overexposure: easy availability, large portions, low prices, prepared food, advertising, subsidizing high-energy food

Technological advances: car, television, computer, remote control, escalator, elevator (each provides valuable benefits, but taken together, they have a cumulative negative effect)

Urban design: zoning restrictions, no destination reachable on foot, lack of pedestrian amenities, lack of bike lanes and trails

Transport options: car dependence, no public transit, lack of safety measures for pedestrians and cyclists

School policies: reduction in physical education classes, exclusivity contracts with soft-drink companies, vending machines filled with snack foods, schools located far from residential areas

22 percent of coronary heart disease, colon cancer, and osteoporotic fractures, 12 percent of diabetes and hypertension, and 5 percent of breast cancer. It accounted for $24.3 billion for direct health-care delivery costs in 1995, or 2.4 percent of U.S. health-care expenditures.[10] Moreover, direct costs for obesity, defined as a body mass index greater than 30, totaled $70 billion in 1995, while indirect costs amounted to at least $48 billion. Physical inactivity in adulthood is also a predictor of disability later in life;

people who are physically inactive during their forties are more likely to have difficulties later in life performing the activities of daily living—such as dressing, rising from a seated position, eating, walking, grooming, reaching, gripping, and doing errands—which compromises their autonomy.[11]

Physical inactivity does not characterize only the American population. In Canada, about two thirds of the population is now physically inactive. The economic burden of this inactivity was estimated for the year 1999; more than $2 billion spent on health care was directly attributable to physical inactivity. This amount represented 2.5 percent of total health-care costs for that year. The total cost attributable to physical inactivity accounted for 25.5 percent of the cost of treating coronary heart disease, stroke, hypertension, colon cancer, breast cancer, type 2 diabetes, and osteoporosis. Moreover, 21,340 premature deaths were also related to physical inactivity. It was estimated that a reduction of 10 percent in the prevalence of physical inactivity would save $150 million per year in health-care costs. The cost of obesity was not included in these calculations.[12]

Among older men and women, bone mineral density at all hip sites is greater in current and lifelong recreational exercisers than in those who engage in mild or no exercise, suggesting a protective effect of exercise on bone mass.[13] Increase in bone mineral density has been related to a lower risk of osteoporotic fracture.

Physical inactivity constitutes an independent risk factor for the development of obesity, so health consequences of a sedentary lifestyle are independent of those associated with obesity. Our energy expenditure has declined because most physical tasks of everyday life are now very limited due to motorized transport, mechanized equipment, and domestic appliances. Labor-saving devices such as lawn mowers, snow-throwers, and leaf-blowers may also contribute to lower physical activity levels, as well as to air pollution. Moreover, the remote control now makes almost any movement unnecessary: a button press by a single finger, and a task that previously required an expenditure of energy is now performed automatically.

Despite a decline in the level of energy intake, obesity is escalating, suggesting that physical inactivity induced by the modern lifestyle plays an important role by itself in the etiology of obesity. Changes in the prevalence of obesity during the second half of the twentieth century even seem to be unrelated to changes in the intake of total energy or of fat; instead, proxy measures of physical inactivity such as car ownership and television viewing were found to be more closely related to changes in the obesity level.[14]

Among fifteen countries of the European Union, it was shown that adults who spent more time sitting down also exercised less in leisure time, were older, were more likely to have gained weight in the past six months, were more often of lower socioeconomic status, and were more likely to be smokers and obese.[15] Data derived from the Pilot Survey of the fitness of Australians also revealed that being too fat was a common barrier to physical activity.[16]

A sedentary lifestyle ranks only behind cigarette smoking and obesity as a contributor to deaths from nine chronic diseases, including coronary heart disease, stroke, and colorectal cancer. According to the CDC, if all physically inactive people became active, we would save $77 billion in annual medical costs.[17]

PHYSICAL INACTIVITY AMONG CHILDREN AND TEENAGERS

Considering that physical activity normally decreases with age, it is worrying to observe its decline even among children. Nearly half of those aged twelve to twenty-one years are not vigorously active on a regular basis,[18] and preschool children spend the majority of their playtime in sedentary activities.

It is now evident that children are exercising less than they were before, in their leisure time and at school as well. Shrinking budgets and an emphasis on academic subjects have led to a reduction in the amount of time devoted to physical education at school. According to the Report of the Surgeon General on physical activity and health in 1996, daily enrollment in physical education classes declined among high school students from 42 percent in 1991 to 25 percent in 1995, just four years later. Illinois was the only state still requiring daily physical education for all class levels in 2003; meanwhile, in Florida, 58 percent of children did not attend gym class in any given week, as reported by ABC News correspondent Geraldine Sealy.[19]

At the same time, looking desperately for funding, schools sign exclusivity contracts with soft-drink companies, allowing them to install vending machines packed with soft drinks and snacks inside the school building. These sweet profits may allow special purchases for the school, but it comes at the expense of student health. It is not the best way to teach children about good nutritional habits and a healthy lifestyle. Rather, these schools are encouraging obesity and the establishment of unhealthy food habits. According to obesity expert Kelly Brownell, who wrote a provocative book about the role of the food industry in the American obesity crisis in 2004,

"Schools do not consider healthy eating relevant to their mission."[20]

It would not be surprising to see these future adults suing the school system for exposing them to unhealthy food habits, as we now see smokers suing tobacco companies. However, one state—California—has become the first to ban soft-drink sales to elementary and junior high school students and to require school-board approval of other junk-food vending contracts; some other states are now following the trend. A study by the Center for Science in the Public Interest found that soft drinks accounted for the ingestion of ten to fifteen teaspoons of sugar per day among teenagers; soft drinks have now exceeded milk as a daily beverage among this age group.[21] The first year that Americans drank more soda than milk was 1976, and they now drink twice as much.[22] Soft drinks are more available than ever before and contribute to excess caloric intake. A study carried out among schoolchildren from four Massachusetts public schools between 1995 and 1997 found that each additional serving of sugar-sweetened drink per day increased the risk of obesity by 60 percent over the nineteen-month period of follow-up.[23]

Because of budget cuts, regular classroom teachers often replace physical education teachers for organizing physical activities, although they are not as qualified to lead them.[24] American children spend less time now in structured physical activities in schools than their European counterparts. When they are engaged in these activities, many of them are standing passively, watching the performance of high-achieving students. Because of the competitive nature of sports, the latter receive the most attention.

In the United Kingdom, the government planned to increase the time spent in physical education classes to reduce the obesity level among children, but the initiative has not had the expected success. Because of their lack of physical fitness and endurance, children fail to meet the required standards. Consequently, many are dropping out of physical education classes, even with the approval of their parents. As the authors of the article observe, they are already "too fat to get fit."[25] The newspaper *The Observer* devoted many articles to the subject in 2003. Schoolchildren do not get enough exercise either at home or at school, and they are also "overfed and dependent on the car," according to the authors. Sports are no longer a priority in the school curriculum; the number of children walking to school is dropping; and sedentary activities such as watching television and computer games are increasingly popular. Parents are more reluctant to let their children play outside because they perceive it as too dangerous.[26,27]

Television viewing and computer games are two important factors involved in the decline of physical activity among children. Because of their importance, they will be reviewed in the next chapter.

Low physical activity was found to be associated with negative health behaviors—such as cigarette smoking, marijuana use, poor dietary habits, excessive television viewing, and failure to wear a seat belt—among a representative sample of U.S. youth.[28]

On the other hand, children with daily physical education sessions during primary school years were found to be more physically active as adults, indicating the long-term positive effect of physical education on exercise habits.[29]

15

The Increase in Obesity

As a nation we are dedicated to keeping physically fit
—and park as close to the stadium as possible.
—*Bill Vaughan*

It is well known that Americans too often eat oversize portions of food, and it is difficult to exercise when you are too full. My first cultural shock about eating practices in the United States occurred in Boston some twenty years ago. I was in a nice restaurant having dinner when I noticed some people leaving with brown paper bags. I thought they had come there to order and were just bringing their takeout meal back home. But when the waiter brought us what we had ordered, I was stunned by the size of the portions. Although we were very hungry, it seemed there was still the same amount of food on our plates at the end of the meal as when we started. So we were asked if we would like "doggy bags" to bring home the leftovers. At first, I thought it was a joke. Then I understood why almost everybody was leaving the restaurant with bags. These oversize portions—and the "all you can eat" practices—have deleterious consequences in the long run.

Excessive food portions have been linked to obesity by researchers. In an experiment carried out by Brian Wansink, a professor at the University of Illinois, the audience at a movie theater was offered free popcorn. Half the group was given fresh popcorn, a small or a large portion. The other half received fourteen-day-old popcorn in small or jumbo containers. Despite the fact that most people who got the old popcorn said it had a terrible taste, those with the bigger portions ate 33 percent more than those with the smaller containers.[1] Similar food experiments have been carried out showing that the more people are given, the more they eat, regardless of whether they are full or the food tastes bad.

Although the worldwide increase in the number of obese people has led to the creation of the concept of "globesity"—more than 1 billion adults are now overweight or obese worldwide—the situation is particularly alarming in North America, as shown in a series of articles published in the *Miami Herald* in June 2003[2] and in a recent edition of *Perspectives in Health: The Magazine of the Pan American Health Organization*.[3] The prevalence of obesity has reached epidemic proportions. Reality does not keep pace any longer with the cultural norm favoring thinness.

The threat of an exploding world population rising far beyond the amount of resources required to sustain it has been surpassed in the last decades by the threat of individual explosion: waistlines are expanding to a degree critical for health concerns.

In 2004, two thirds of American adults were overweight or obese, according to statistics from the CDC. One of three adults was overweight, with a body-mass index between 25 and 30 kg/m^2; another one of three was obese according to the World Health Organization definition, which means having a body-mass index over 30 kg/m^2. In 1991, the proportion of overweight people was 45 percent, while the prevalence of obesity was 12 percent.[4] A steady increase was observed in all states, in both sexes, and across all age groups, races, and educational levels, and regardless of smoking status. A higher prevalence was found in eastern and southern states. The greatest increase was seen, alarmingly, among eighteen- to twenty-nine-year-olds.[5] These proportions are probably underestimated because they are based on self-reported weight and height. Nevertheless, obesity prevalence increased by 61 percent between 1991 and 2000.

Some 15 million American adults over the age of fifty-one were obese in 2003, according to the Center on an Aging Society at Georgetown University in Washington, D.C. These adults were twice as likely to have difficulty with multiple activities of daily living, were more likely to suffer from chronic symptoms of illness such as fatigue, wheezing, and shortness of breath, and to report feelings of sadness and hopelessness. Obesity was also shown to affect their lifestyle by reducing their ability to participate in activities such as walking, shopping, and attending movies, parties, or other social events. Also, they were more likely to miss work because of health problems.[6]

THE CASE OF EXTREME OBESITY

An analysis from the Rand Corporation revealed that extreme obesity (being at least 100 pounds overweight or having a body-mass index of at least 40) affected 4 million American adults in 2000; in 1986, it was the case for 1 in 200 adults, while in 2000 the proportion reached 1 in 50.[7] The proportion of morbidly obese persons has increased even faster than the proportion of obese people with a body-mass index between 30 and 40. Morbid obesity incurs the highest health-care costs.

OBESITY REDUCES LONGEVITY

Obesity affects longevity as well. Data from the famous Framingham Heart Study, which followed more than 5,000 adults from 1948 to 1990, indicated large decreases in life expectancy among overweight or obese people at baseline: a forty-year-old overweight nonsmoker lived three years less than a nonsmoker with a normal weight. For obese participants, the difference was many years greater.[8] Lifespan between 1971 and 1999 was found to be higher among adults having an optimal body-mass index between 23 and 25 for whites and between 23 and 30 for blacks, still showing that overweight and obesity reduce life expectancy.[9] From there, considering the skyrocketing obesity among the new generations, combined with their low level of physical activity, it would not be surprising to observe an overall decrease of population life expectancy in the near future.

OBESITY AMONG CHILDREN

One in seven American children is now obese, which means five million of them. More than 15 percent of teenagers were overweight in 1999–2000, according to the National Health and Nutrition Examination Survey, which also showed an increase in the prevalence of overweight among American children between 1988 and 1994 and between 1999 and 2000. The prevalence of overweight rose from 7.2 percent to 10.4 percent among two- to five-year-olds, from 11.3 percent to 15.3 percent among six- to eleven-year-olds, and from 10.5 percent to 15.5 percent among twelve- to nineteen-year-olds.[10] While physical education was often left aside in schools because of budget cuts, or priority given to more academic subjects, fast-food companies were making their entrance, feeding more and more children with French fries, pizza, and soft drinks at lunchtime and thus molding their future food habits. In 2002, the British medical journal *Lancet* reported childhood obesity as a public-health crisis worldwide because of the many countries affected by the devastating trend, from the United States to England, China, Japan, and Australia, as well as many developing countries.[11]

Because of its long-term adverse consequences, obesity in early childhood is particularly alarming. According to the Feeding Infants and Toddlers Study published in the January 2004 edition of the *Journal of the American Dietetic Association*, improper eating habits start very early in life, even before age two. In this survey, up to one third of the children under two years consumed no fruits or vegetables, and among those who ate vegetables, French fries were the most common item for children fifteen months and older, while hot dogs, sausage, and bacon were part of the daily staples for 25 percent of the older group.[12] Children between one and two years of age were found to have an excess energy intake of nearly 30 percent: their median intake was 1,220 calories, whereas the requirements for that age are about 950 calories per day. These findings are really troubling, considering the fact that food preferences and overeating habits are shaped very early in life. Moreover, children of obese parents are more likely to be obese themselves, as revealed by Statistics Canada.

Severe obesity can be psychologically devastating among children and adolescents. The likelihood of having an impaired health–related quality of life, based on physical, emotional, social, and school functioning, has been found to be 5.5 times greater in a severely obese child or adolescent than in one who is healthy, similar to those diagnosed with cancer.[13] An experiment carried out for ABC News for its special *Fat Like Me* in October 2003 also stressed the psychological impact of obesity: a slim teenage girl padded and layered with latex to make her look as though she weighed 200 pounds was laughed at by other kids when she entered a new high school; she found this one-day experience excruciating.[14] Even though there are more obese children now than ever, they are still stigmatized because the social norm requires being slim and good-looking.

AN EXCESSIVE CALORIC INTAKE

An increase in the prevalence of obesity has occurred despite the dramatic rise in the percentage of the American population consuming low-calorie products, which went from 19 percent in 1978 to 76 percent in 1991, illustrating the failure of this weight-control strategy.[15] Added to this failure is the disturbing fact that less than half of obese persons who had had a routine checkup in the preceding year were advised by health-care professionals to lose weight. Among those who were trying to lose or maintain weight, only 17.5 percent were following recommendations to eat fewer calories and increase physical activity to more than 150 minutes per week.[16]

Most people do not eat enough fresh fruits and vegetables—the recommended five portions per day—despite their easy availability, preferring to rely on ready-to-serve meals. The price of produce may be a deterrent to higher consumption. As shown by *Consumer Reports*, the consumer price of fresh fruits and vegetables increased by 127 percent between 1982 and 2003, while at the same time the price of fats and oils rose only 57 percent, ground beef fattened on cheap grains 50 percent, and soft drinks 26 percent. According to this magazine, the main reason is that each year in America the federal government pays $20 billion to subsidize the production of rice, soybeans, sugar, wheat, and corn, but no such subsidy program exists for fruits and vegetables. This has led, for example, to skyrocketing consumption of corn syrup, which has multiplied by forty times over the last twenty years.[17] High-fructose corn syrup is used as a sweetener for a huge variety of foods. In subsidizing these high-calorie foods, the government is sending the wrong message to the population, encouraging obesity and the resulting diabetes epidemic.

It is also suspected that some foods such as cheese contain natural constituents called opioids which could be addictive, encouraging people to eat more of them and even become addicted. This may explain why cheese is one of the most difficult items to avoid for people who are dieting or for those becoming vegans.[18]

THE FAILURE OF DIETS

More than one third of American adults are now trying to lose weight, and nearly the same proportion are trying to maintain their present weight.[19] Nearly five million American adults—or 2.5 percent of the adult population—used prescription weight-loss pills between 1996 and 1998, even though one quarter of them were not even overweight.[20] Considering the proportions of overweight and obese people, these solutions do not seem very efficient.

CHECK YOUR OWN BMI

Many people do not have an accurate perception of their weight. Some think they are overweight when they are not, and others believe they are in the normal range, despite an obvious weight surplus. Here is how to calculate your BMI (body mass index) and find out where you really stand.

BMI = weight (in kilograms) ÷ height² (in meters)

To find your weight in kilograms, multiply your weight in pounds by 0.454; to find your height in meters, multiply your height in inches by 0.025. For example, if you weigh 165 pounds, your weight in kilograms is 74.9; if you are 71 inches tall (5 feet, 11 inches), your height in meters is 1.8.

So if you weigh 75 kg and you are 1.8 meters tall, then your BMI is:

75 ÷ (1.8 x 1.8) = 23.1

A BMI between 18 and 25 is considered normal; a BMI between 25 and 30 indicates overweight, and over 30 indicates obesity.

OBESE CITIES AND COUNTRIES

Every year, *Men's Fitness* magazine publishes a list of the twenty-five fattest cities and the twenty-five fittest ones. According to the lists for 2003, the fattest cities were Detroit, Houston, Dallas, San Antonio, and Chicago, while the top fittest were Honolulu, San Francisco, Virginia Beach, Denver, and Colorado Springs.[21] The fact that Detroit, the city of automobiles, ranked first is another indication of the relationship between the built environment and obesity. It is not very easy to walk in this city. The state of Texas accounted for five of the top ten fattest cities, despite the high availability there of fresh fruits and vegetables. Most of these cities are characterized by sprawl, where distances are too long to be covered on foot. In this ranking, the cities were rated on fourteen categories, including gyms and sporting goods, nutrition, junk-food restaurants, exercise and sports participation, overweight and sedentary life, alcohol consumption, television watching, air quality, climate, access to outdoor recreation, commuting time, parks and open space, recreational facilities, and access to health-care facilities.

Although this kind of ranking may not be based on a scientific analysis according to the experts, it nevertheless reflects large differences in the quality of the urban environment from one city to another, and in the obesity rates of their residents.

The United States is not the only country to show an alarming obesity rate. Australia is also strongly affected by the epidemic: according to the 1999–2000 Australian Diabetes, Obesity and Lifestyle Study, the prevalence of overweight and obesity in both sexes (defined by either BMI or waist circumference) was almost 60 percent, which is 2.5 times higher than in 1980.[22] Up north in Canada, the prevalence of obesity in children aged seven to thirteen years more than doubled between 1981 and 1996, going from 5 percent to 13.5 percent for boys and 11.8 percent for girls.[23] According to an article in an August 2003 issue of *Time* magazine, 10 percent of Chinese children were said to be overweight (i.e., 30 million), and the number could double in a decade.[24]

In the meantime, overweight and obesity are less common in most European countries, although the problem is on the rise over there too, especially in the U.K. and Germany.[25] Scandinavian countries such as Norway and Finland have already taken drastic measures to change the high-fat, energy-dense diet of their populations and have been able to reduce cholesterol levels and the number of deaths from coronary heart disease.[26]

The dramatic increase in overweight and obesity is not all attributable to energy intake but also to physical inactivity, encouraged by environmental influences.[27] After visiting San Antonio, Texas, in 2003, the health editor of the British newspaper *The Guardian* called this city "the fat capital of the world." He noticed that in addition to the oversized portions in restaurants, it was difficult to walk anywhere because the blocks were too long and the roads too wide.[28] The prevalence of obesity has been found to be more strongly related to lower levels of physical activity than to higher energy intake.[29] Two economists of the Rand Corporation attributed 60 percent of the rise in obesity rates over the past two decades to sedentary jobs, and 40 percent to the availability of cheap, plentiful food.[30]

Almost everything in our environment promotes physical inactivity, and this problem is much more common in North America than in Europe. As pointed out recently by a reader of the special January 2004 health and fitness edition of *Consumer Reports*,[31] "Government policies promote the shifting of corporate costs to tax-payers through road-building gasoline taxes, and to employees through increasing commute times and driving costs, thus contributing to making America a more unhealthful place to live and work." This resident of San Diego reported that he had involuntarily lost more than thirty pounds living in the Paris area (France) for six months several years ago, because he did not have a car and had to rely upon his feet and what he called the "best mass-transit system in the world" for transportation.[32]

16

Obesity and Health

To say that obesity is caused by merely consuming
too many calories is like saying that the only cause of the
American Revolution was the Boston Tea Party.

—*Adelle Davis (American nutritionist and writer)*

Obesity also has a huge impact on all kind of diseases: coronary heart disease, hypertension, high blood cholesterol, type 2 diabetes, osteoarthritis, cancer, musculoskeletal disorders, sleep apnea, and gall bladder disease.[1,2] Moreover, it was recently found to be a risk factor for dementia, and more particularly Alzheimer's disease, among older women in Sweden.[3] Not only obesity, but also overweight was found to increase the risk of developing gallstones, hypertension, high cholesterol, and heart disease in both sexes.[4]

Obese people are not only sicker, they are also at greater risk of developing diseases, which suggests a causal relationship between obesity and the occurrence of disease. A ten-year follow-up of a cohort of more than 120,000 participants in the Nurses' Health Study and the Health Professionals Follow-up Study showed a higher incidence of diabetes, hypertension, gallstones, heart disease, and stroke among those who were overweight at the beginning of the study in 1986; the risk increased with the severity of overweight.[5] According to the American Medical Association, almost 80 percent of obese adults have diabetes, high blood cholesterol, high blood pressure, coronary artery disease, gallbladder disease, or osteoarthritis, and almost 40 percent have two or more of these.[6]

It is now suspected that obesity also has adverse effects on brain function.

TEN LEADING HEALTH PROBLEMS LINKED TO OBESITY

There is a debate about how many deaths are attributable to obesity each year. But beyond the exact number of deaths, it is widely recognized that obesity carries its own ailments. Among the most common are:

- Type 2 diabetes
- High blood cholesterol
- Hypertension
- Cardiovascular disease
- Almost all types of cancer
- Osteoarthritis
- Musculoskeletal disorders
- Sleep apnea
- Gallbladder disease
- Depression

Research based on follow-up of participants in the famous Framingham Heart Study recently found a relationship between obesity, hypertension, and cognitive performance in late-middle-aged and elderly men, independent of other common cardiovascular risk factors: obese and hypertensive men performed more poorly on learning, executive functioning, and abstract reasoning. The two factors were independently related to cognitive performance. The underlying process is thought to be that excess fat affects blood circulation in the brain, increasing the risk of ministrokes and hemorrhages that can cause a decline in mental functioning.[7]

Health economist Roland Sturm of the Rand Corporation compared the effects of obesity, smoking, and drinking on the occurrence of chronic health conditions and health-care expenditures in a national survey of adults aged eighteen to sixty-five years carried out in 1997–1998. The results, published in the April 2002 issue of the medical journal *Health Affairs,* showed that the effects of obesity on the occurrence of chronic conditions were larger than the effects of current or past smoking or problem drinking, and treatment costs for health care and medication were also greater. The effects of obesity were similar to those of twenty years' aging. The author believed his results could only be the tip of the iceberg, since most of the long-term consequences of increased obesity have not yet appeared.[8]

OVERSIZED HOSPITAL EQUIPMENT

The increase in obesity has required hospitals to equip themselves with heavy-duty medical supplies and to design plus-sized rooms, as reported in the January 13, 2004, *Chicago Sun-Times*.[9] Hospitals now need scales that tip 1,000 pounds, reinforced toilets, oversized beds, wheelchairs that can carry two normal-sized adults, and blood pressure cuffs as big as thighs. Nationwide, 17 percent of hospitals say they have had to remodel to accommodate severely obese people. Novation, a group-purchasing organization for hospitals and other health-care institutions, quoted 80 percent of hospitals in its survey as saying they had treated more severely obese patients in the last year than ever before. Some hospitals estimate additional costs associated with treating or accommodating the severely obese can reach up to $500,000 per year per institution. According to the CDC, care for overweight and obese patients costs an average of 37 percent more than for people of normal weight, adding an average of $732 to the annual medical bill of every American.[10]

OBESITY AND QUALITY OF LIFE

A poorer quality of life in older age was recently found related to overweight and obesity, after following for twenty-six years a cohort of nearly 7,000 middle-aged men and women from the Chicago Heart Association Detection Project in Industry. Normal-weight individuals had better health status physically, emotionally, and socially. In comparison with overweight individuals, a higher proportion of those of normal weight had no limitation in common physical activities, which indicates that not only disease but also a person's entire quality of life can be compromised by having a higher-than-recommended body-mass index.[11]

CHILDREN'S HEALTH

Early signs of heart disease have been found among overweight American children, as reported by *NewScientist* in November 2003.[12] About one million of them now suffer from a condition called metabolic syndrome, which makes them more prone to type 2 diabetes and premature heart disease. The risk factors associated with this syndrome include high blood pressure, excessive abdominal fat, high triglyceride levels, low levels of good cholesterol, and high blood sugar. A study conducted by the School of Nursing of the University of North Carolina at Chapel Hill on 3,200 children in rural North Carolina found the presence of three or more risk factors in about one in seven schoolchildren; girls were particularly at risk, being 50 percent more likely to have three risk factors. The most common risk factor, seen in 42 percent of the group, was low levels of good cholesterol. Children with type 2 diabetes are more likely to develop heart disease in their twenties and thirties.[13]

OBESITY AND DISABILITY

As a risk factor for osteoarthritis, obesity is also responsible for disability, leading to days in bed, work days lost, and restricted activity days. Part of the reason is increased pressure on the joints in overweight persons. It is also related to mobility limitations.[14] Using data from the National Health Interview Survey, researchers from the Rand Corporation showed an increase in the rate of disability between 1984 and 2000 among people aged eighteen to fifty-nine, especially among those between thirty and forty-nine years, where the rates increased by more than 50 percent. During the same period, disability declined by more than 10 percent for people aged sixty to sixty-nine years. The authors of the study suggest a link between the emerging growth of disability among younger groups and the increase in obesity, which could entail adverse consequences for public health programs. The number of disability cases attributed to musculoskeletal problems and diabetes grew more rapidly than those from other problems; diabetes-related disability alone doubled between 1984 and 2000. Disability rates are rising for whites and nonwhites, for people inside and outside the labor force, and for all education groups.[15]

OBESITY AND CANCER

Too much body fat increases the amount of estrogen in the blood, raising the risk of cancers of the female reproductive system. It also increases the risk of acid reflux, which can cause cancer of the esophagus, and it raises levels of insulin, prompting the body to create a hormone which causes cells to multiply. A possible mechanism discussed by the World Cancer Research Fund for the relationship between high body weight and cancer relates to the metabolic abnormalities resulting from high body-mass-index levels; these abnormalities promote cell growth and especially growth of tumor cells.[16]

A recent study was published in the *Journal of the American Medical Association* that followed a cohort of 900,000 American adults over sixteen years (from 1982 to 1998); 57,000 deaths from cancer occurred during this period, and the authors showed that overweight contributed to cancers of the breast, uterus, ovary, cervix, colon, rectum, kidney, esophagus, gall bladder, and pancreas, multiple myeloma, non-Hodgkin's lymphoma, and cancers of the liver, stomach, and prostate. The heaviest members of the cohort (with a body mass index of at least 40 kg/m²) had death rates from all cancers 52 percent higher in men and 62 percent higher in women than those of normal weight. Based on these calculations, overweight might account for 14 percent of all cancer deaths in men and 20 percent of those in women fifty years of age or older. According to these results, losing weight to maintain a body-mass index below 25 kg/m² throughout life could prevent 90,000 deaths each year in the United States.[17] And this is only for cancer!

THE DIABETES EPIDEMIC

Obesity is the most important risk factor for type 2 diabetes, which is skyrocketing worldwide. In the United States alone, 1.3 million cases were diagnosed in 2002. Obese people are five to ten times more likely to suffer from the disease than those of normal weight. The prevalence of type 2 diabetes went from 4.9 percent of the adult population in 1990 to 7.3 percent in 2000—that is nearly 15 million adults eighteen years of age or older.[18] Forty-three U.S. states had diabetes rates 6 percent or greater in 2000, compared to four states in 1990; the lowest rates were found in Alaska, Idaho, Montana, New Hampshire, Vermont, Nebraska, and Oklahoma, while the highest were in Alabama, California, Maryland, Mississippi, and South Carolina. The numbers were even higher after adding the undiagnosed diabetes cases, as reported by the Centers for Disease Control and Prevention;[19] the total would then be 29 million persons aged twenty years and older. In El Paso, Texas, the rate of diabetes has reached 12.9 percent and is clearly linked to the high prevalence of overweight and obesity in the city. Not coincidentally, Houston is also characterized by urban sprawl development, where walking and biking are not easy and public transportation is limited.[20]

In Australia, the prevalence of diabetes was found to be 7.4 percent in 2000, more than twice the estimate for 1981, now one of the highest rates in the industrialized world.[21]

Diabetes is the most expensive public-health consequence of obesity.[22] Concentrations of free fatty acids, which increase insulin resistance, are excessive in individuals with abdominal obesity. According to the World Health Organization, about 64 percent of type 2 diabetes in U.S. men and 74 percent in U.S. women could be avoided if people kept their body mass indexes below 25 kg/m².[23]

Once an adult disease, type 2 diabetes is now common among children. According to the CDC, a child born in 2000 has more than one chance in three of developing type 2 diabetes during his or her lifetime; the highest life-time risk is among Hispanics, where it reaches nearly 50 percent.[24] The disease is also more common among African-Americans and Native Americans than among Caucasians. In China, diabetes is becoming very common in cities, where the economic boom has led to rapid changes in diet and lifestyle.

Diabetes is a disease of affluence. According to the "thrifty gene" theory developed by geneticist James Neel in 1962, the disease is linked to past human evolution, when it was advantageous to have genes promoting slow metabolism and storage of fat because it helped our ancestors survive the frequent and unpredictable periods of famine. Those who had such a thrifty gene were more likely to survive and pass it on to their descendants. They may have developed diseases related to obesity later on, but only after the reproductive period was over. In modern society, in which food is always plentiful and very cheap, the same gene contributes to insulin resistance, obesity, and diabetes. Because the environment and the circumstances have changed, "the thrifty gene is an asset that becomes a liability," according to Jared Diamond, an evolutionary biologist and Pulitzer Prize winner working at the University of California at Los Angeles. Diamond published an article on the thrifty gene in the British journal *Nature* in 2003. As he mentions, the ability to store fat and burn it slowly was "an accommodation to the pendulum of feast and famine that was very necessary in times when that pendulum swung often but irregularly—a situation that was much more typical of our evolutionary history than the state of plenty to which we are accustomed."[25]

People with diabetes are more likely to develop heart disease. But, as reported in *Time* in the issue of December 8, 2003, this condition also damages small blood vessels throughout the body, particularly in the eyes and kidneys, leading to blindness. In the United States, 24,000 diabetics become blind each year, while more than 100,000 require dialysis or kidney transplantation; and 82,000 need amputations.[26] They are also twice as likely as nondiabetics to suffer from depression.

OBESITY AND MORTALITY

A poor diet and physical inactivity were responsible for 400,000 deaths in the United States in 2000, just slightly behind tobacco, which is still the number-one killer. The rapid increase in the prevalence of overweight suggests that it may soon overtake tobacco as the leading cause of death.[27]

The relationship between obesity and all-cause mortality is more pronounced in white than in black people—although the latter are more prone to overweight—and it is stronger among those who have never smoked than among smokers.[28] Obesity now stands second, right behind smoking, among the leading causes of death. Deaths linked to obesity have been found to shorten life by nine years on average.[29] Data from six studies revealed that more than 80 percent of the estimated deaths attributable to obesity occurred among individuals with a body-mass index of more than 30kg/m^2, and the number of annual deaths attributable to obesity was 280,184, according to an analysis carried out by the Obesity Research Center in New York.[30]

THE SPREAD OF OBESITY TO OUR PETS

The obesity problem is spreading to our beloved pets as well, as reported in the *San Matteo Times* in California in December 2003.[31] A decade ago, 15 percent of pets were overweight; the proportion is now around 40 percent, because the pets have adopted the sedentary lifestyle and food habits of their owners. Dogs do not exercise enough because their owners do not take them out often or long enough. Moreover, the same owners have difficulty limiting the food intake of their pets, although the animals would live 15 percent longer if they had a normal weight.

According to the nation's largest provider of pet health insurance (more than 350,000 policyholders), there was a tremendous rise in claims for diabetes, hypertension, and even cardiac arrest for dogs and cats in the last few years. Pets are often seen as a mirror of their owners; what happens to them should be a warning signal for humans. A similar trend toward a diabetes epidemic was observed among the captive primate species of the Los Angeles Zoo by Jared Diamond while he was on the Animal Regulation Committee. The lifestyle of these animals mimics the high-calorie, low-exercise lifestyle of North Americans.[32]

TO THE RESCUE OF SEDENTARY DOGS

Some organizations, like PAWS (Providence Animal Walking and Sitting), are very concerned with the level of physical inactivity among dogs these days. Their message is: "Don't let your dog get sad, lazy, and overweight. Call us to walk your dog while you are out." This tactful message suggests how sedentary some dog owners are, but unfortunately, the adverse consequences are not just for the animal.

17

The Costs of Obesity

Addiction, obesity, starvation (anorexia nervosa) are political
problems, not psychiatric: each condenses and expresses a contest
between the individual and some other person or persons in his
environment over the control of the individual's body.

—*Thomas Szasz (American psychiatrist)*

Direct costs of obesity totaled $70 billion in 1995, or 7 percent of national health-care expenditures in the United States, and indirect costs amount to at least $48 billion, the major contributor being coronary heart disease, which accounts for a large percentage of premature mortality.[1] The cost of lost productivity attributed to obesity was $3.9 billion in 1994, reflecting 39.2 million days of lost work. Added to this, 239 million restricted-activity days, 89.5 million bed-days, and 62.6 million physician visits were attributable to obesity in 1994.[2] The number of physician visits attributed to obesity increased 88 percent from 1988 to 1994.

In 1996, there were 9.3 million cases of cardiovascular disease among obese people, almost half of them associated with obesity, leading to $22.2 billion in direct medical costs, 17 percent of the total direct medical cost of treating this problem.[3]

Direct costs of diabetes were estimated to be $92 billion in 2002, while indirect costs reached $40 billion, making diabetes the most expensive consequence of obesity.[4] These costs now account for 15 percent of health-care costs in the United States and have reached $100 billion.[5] Pharmaceuticals also account for a substantial share of costs attributable to obesity. Worldwide, the cost of drug treatment for diabetes alone was estimated at as much as $12 billion in 2002.[6]

Personal costs are not included in these estimations. Job discrimination related to the stigma associated with obesity, or to diseases and disabilities caused by it, higher premiums from insurance companies, and limitations in daily life also impair the condition of obese people, but calculations of the costs involved are not easily done.[7] In its September 21, 2003, issue, *The Boston Globe* reported on workplace prejudice against the overweight, noting that it is as prevalent as it was ten years ago, despite the general increase in American waistlines.[8]

In Canada, the direct cost of obesity in 1997 was estimated to be over $1.8 billion, accounting for 2.4 percent of total health-care expenditures; the three largest contributors were hypertension, type 2 diabetes, and coronary heart disease.[9]

Added to health-care costs are obesity-attributable business expenditures on paid sick leave, life insurance, and disability insurance. For 1994, these costs were estimated to be $5 billion for the U.S. economy.[10]

OBESITY AND FITNESS IN THE MILITARY

The consequences of physical inactivity and obesity may soon reach sectors of life we would not have thought of before. As a large part of the general population has become overweight and unfit, and at a much younger age than before, it could become harder for the military to recruit young men and women with the required fitness level to defend the country, especially if conscription were to become necessary. Under such circumstances, the high prevalence of obesity and physical inactivity could constitute a threat to national security, the troops being "too fat to fight."

It was recently found that a significant proportion of American young adults do not meet the weight standards of the military forces, overweight being higher among blacks and Hispanics, who are numerous in the U.S. Army.[11] Overweight is also more common among lower socioeconomic classes, from which more candidates are recruited. Some disturbing trends recently emerged. A vast study of physical activity patterns among military service members stationed at thirty-eight large installations revealed that less than two-thirds exercised three times a week for fifteen to twenty minutes, and 15 percent did not exercise at all, which is not very encouraging.[12] Diabetes was as frequent in the Army as in the general population, where it has reached a critical level.[13] Among active-duty Air Force personnel, total excess costs attributable to body weight were estimated at $22.8 million per year, for medical care and workdays lost.[14]

18

The Role of Television

*If it weren't for the fact that the TV set and the refrigerator
are so far apart, some of us wouldn't get any exercise at all.*
                    —Joey Adams

TV WATCHING AND SOCIAL LIFE

Television viewing has strongly contributed to the American sedentary lifestyle, and this activity has been continuously increasing. Following sleep and work, it is now the third most time-consuming activity. In 2000, 76 percent of American households had more than one television set, and 41 percent had three or more, while 85 percent owned a VCR.[1] Watching TV is the top leisure-time activity among adults; the American adult now watches TV around four hours a day. In 1995, television absorbed 40 percent of the average American's free time.[2] The TV set occupies the dominant place in the family room, and family life revolves around it. It has been shown that couples spend three or four times as much time watching television together as they spend talking to each other. As Robert Putnam points out in his book *Bowling Alone*, watching things occupies more and more of our time, while doing things (especially with others) occupies less and less.[3] Even talking with each other is compromised by television. It decreases the close ties of family life based on oral communication; turning on a television is enough to reduce a room full of people to silence.[4] Instead of participants, they become witnesses of other actors, and the stage has been removed from their life to someone else's.

As the number of TV sets per household increases, more people are watching television alone.[5] And children now spend more time in front of the TV than in school or in direct communication with their parents. Television watching is a big part of the cocooning process: it keeps us home, comfortably watching what is going on in the outside world, and leaving us with less time for socializing outside the home. It has also become an individualized activity rather than an activity promoting family togetherness. Even among children, more than one-third of TV watching is done alone. Moreover, half of Americans report watching television while eating dinner. The high number of available channels has made channel surfing an activity in itself.

Beyond becoming a more individualized activity, television viewing was shown by Robert Putnam to be linked to civic disengagement.[6] Civic participation and social involvement were reduced as TV watching increased. In his study of the rise of civic disengagement in the United States, Putnam has demonstrated how television viewing is incompatible with a major commitment to community life.

Robert Putnam reported that people who say TV is their primary form of entertainment volunteer and work on community projects less often, socialize less, and are less interested in politics than others; they also give blood less often and express more road rage. Putnam reports that television dependence is associated with less involvement in community life, but also with less social communication in all its forms—oral, written, or electronic. As he explains, it is not because heavy TV viewers do not have time for social activities. Comparing them with people who spend a lot of time reading newspapers, for example, he found the latter more engaged in social activities; heavy reading was linked to group membership and social trust, while heavy TV viewing was not. "TV watching comes at the expense of nearly every social activity outside the home, especially social gatherings and informal conversations," he notes. Putnam found heavy television viewing associated with lots of free time, loneliness, and emotional difficulties.[7]

One possible explanation for the impact of television watching on social participation, Putnam suggests, is that television encourages passivity and lethargy, while at the same time providing a pseudo–personal connection to others, giving the individual the feeling of personally knowing the people seen on the screen. It creates a false sense of companionship, making people feel they are engaged without the necessity of any real commitment. The psychological impact of the medium itself has a negative effect on civic participation.

TV WATCHING AND HEALTH

According to some British researchers, excessive television viewing may encourage both sloth and gluttony (the "couch potato effect").[8] Television viewing reduces energy expenditure through its effects on metabolic rate; and because it decreases the time available for more vigorous activities, it facilitates weight gain, which is reinforced by exposure to food advertising on television. In 1997, fast-food restaurants spent over 95 percent of their advertising budgets on TV commercials, and food manufacturers, retailers, and food services spent $11 billion on mass-media advertising. The foods that are most heavily advertised are also those that are overconsumed.[9] Snacking in front of the TV has become a common habit; it may lead to overeating, because people pay less attention to the amounts or types of food they consume while watching television than when they are at the table during mealtimes.[10] Responding to a case study of unhealthy food and leisure habits among an obese family of four reported in the *Las Vegas Review-Journal,* many pediatric experts said children who eat while watching television consume more calories and are more likely to be overweight or obese.[11]

It is easy to understand why television watching is associated with measures of adiposity and excess weight or obesity among people of all ages. Men and women who watched TV more than three hours per day were twice as likely to be obese as those who watched TV for less than one hour, even after controlling for age, smoking status, weekly hours of exercise, and length of work week.[12,13] This phenomenon is not exclusive to Americans; in Australia, adults watching more than four hours of television per day were four times more likely to be overweight than those watching television less than one hour. Body-mass index and physical activity patterns were both associated with amount of television watching.[14,15]

The time spent watching television has also been found to be associated with the occurrence of type 2 diabetes among a cohort of American adults, including 68,500 women and 37,900 men. In women, each two-hour increment in TV watching was associated with a 23 percent increase in the risk of diabetes; the association persisted after adjustment for body-mass index.[16,17]

TV WATCHING AMONG CHILDREN

The main concern about the relationship between television watching and obesity is nevertheless for younger age groups. As noted, children spend more time in front of the TV than in school or in direct interaction with their parents.[18] At the same time, there is an epidemic of childhood overweight and obesity.

Data collected from more than 13,000 children and adolescents in the National Health Examination Survey show an association between the time spent watching television and the prevalence of obesity, even after controlling for other factors such as prior obesity, region, season, race, population density, socioeconomic class, and many family variables; the prevalence of obesity increased 2 percent for each hour of television watched per day.[19] A strong dose-response relationship was also observed in 1990 between the prevalence of overweight and hours of television watching among children ten to fifteen years old: those watching more than five hours of television per day (one third of the sample) had a 4.6 times greater chance of being overweight compared to those watching none to two hours, even after adjustment for overweight at baseline, gender, poverty, mother's ethnicity, education, marital status, and employment.[20]

Data from the National Health and Nutrition Examination Survey III reveal that in 1994, 26 percent of American children aged eight to sixteen years watched four or more hours of television per day, and 67 percent watched at least two hours per day; the highest prevalence of heavy watching occurred among eleven-to-thirteen-year-old children. The survey showed an association between adiposity and television viewing.[21]

Among U.S. high school students, data from the 1999 national Youth Risk Behavior Survey reveal that television viewing on an average school day exceeds two hours among 43 percent of students; the proportion was greater among black (74 percent) and Hispanic (52 percent) than white (34 percent) students. Watching TV more than two hours per day was associated with being overweight in all groups, except black and Hispanic males.[22]

Of particular concern is the fact that the relationship between TV watching and overweight or obesity is already present between four and six years old, which is a period where body fatness usually reaches its lowest level.[23]

Three mechanisms might explain how television viewing relates to obesity. Television watching reduces the resting metabolic rate, thus decreasing total energy expenditure; children spending hours in front of the TV daily have less time left to engage in more energetic activities; and there is increased caloric consumption while watching TV (the snacking habit), probably the effect of food advertising.[24,25] Food is the most heavily advertised product on children's television.[26] At the beginning of 2004, the Kaiser Family Foundation published a report on the role of media in childhood obesity. Reviewing the studies on the subject, the report showed that children now spend an average of 5.5 hours a day using media—including television, videos, video games, and computers—and are then exposed to extensive advertising campaigns. A special edition of ABC News's *PrimeTime Live* was devoted to this subject on December 8, 2003. The journalists reported that the food industry spends $12 billion per year advertising food to this young audience on television, and most of the ads are for processed and unhealthy junk food. The average American child is bombarded with 10,000 food ads each year. Exposure to food advertising is believed to influence children's food choices and requests for products in the supermarket. Some countries have already taken actions to protect children from the intense marketing of food companies. For instance, food advertisement to children under twelve is forbidden in Norway and Sweden; not surprisingly, it happens that these countries also show lower overall obesity rates compared to the rest of the world.[27]

Many children now have a TV set in their bedrooms. Among sixth-graders, the proportion went from 6 percent in 1970 to 77 percent in 1999.[28] In a study carried out in New York state among low-income families, it was found that 40 percent of children younger than five years had a television in their bedrooms; they were more likely to be overweight and spent more time watching than those without a TV in their bedrooms.[29] A report of the Kaiser Family Foundation dealing with television habits among children six months to six years old revealed that young children living in homes where the television is on most of the time may have more trouble learning to read.

Children begin to watch TV at a very young age. The National Longitudinal Survey of Youth, 1990 to 1998, studied television viewing from birth to thirty-five months of age and followed the trajectory of a child's viewing from infancy through age six. The parents of 17 percent of children up to eleven months old, 48 percent of children twelve to twenty-three months old, and 41 percent of children twenty-four to thirty-five months old reported more television watching among their children than the American Academy of Pediatrics recommends (no television before age two, and less than two hours per day for children two years and older).[30]

Why so much television watching among children? Their parents also watch more television than before, but this is not the only reason. Children spend less time outside the home without supervision than a few decades ago. In many areas, the parents consider it unsafe to let children play outside by themselves, and they do not have enough time to supervise them. Despite the high availability of toys and games of all kinds, children spend less time playing and developing their imaginations than watching television. More of them are only children than in the past. In the United States, the percentage of women who have only one child has more than doubled in the past twenty years, up from 10 percent to over 23 percent. One-child families are the fastest-growing group of families. There are now an estimated twenty million only-child households in the United States (see www.onlychild.com/aboutus/letter.html). Lacking siblings to play with, the only child relies on television for companionship and imagination; and for the child's parents, the TV set often acts as a baby-sitter substitute, supervising the child's activities and keeping him or her quiet while the parents are too busy to do so.

While researching information on television and obesity among children, I was surprised to find an unexpected health hazard: television sets toppling over onto children cause serious and sometimes fatal injuries. Between 1990 and 1997, seventy-three cases in which a TV set fell on a child were reported to the Consumer Product Safety Commission; in twenty-eight of these, the child was killed. Head injuries were the most common occurrence. The mean age of those who died was thirty-one months.[31,32]

19
A Suburban Scenario

*Suburbia is where the developer bulldozes
out the trees, then names the streets after them.*
—*Bill Vaughan*

It is a very nice neighborhood at first sight, extremely clean and quiet, only single homes for wealthy families—a residential area not reached by the agitation of daily life, except when its residents leave in the morning and come back home after work. No workplaces, stores, schools, or restaurants bring noise and strangers into the vicinity. Most of the time, there is nobody outside. In any case, there is no place to go on foot, and the cul-de-sac (dead-end) street pattern makes it harder to reach any destination. At rush hour pedestrians are not allowed on the streets, both for their own safety and because they can disturb the traffic flow. To allow wider streets, no sidewalks were built. The back yard is the only accessible safe area. At any other time, pedestrians have to wear walking helmets to reduce their risk of head injury; since safety campaigns were not convincing enough, helmet wearing is now mandatory. On busy streets, a breathing mask is also required to protect humans from traffic air-pollution. The level of respiratory diseases became so high that municipal authorities had to find a drastic solution to reduce the problem. Wearing a mask became a normal habit after the SARS epidemic a few years earlier. As a safety measure, walking on the streets has been prohibited from dusk to dawn.

Brian and Tracy moved here ten years ago with their young family. Because it was so quiet and filled with young families, they thought it would be the perfect location to raise their two children, Tim and Laura, although they have to commute to work about one hour each twice a day, and not in the same direction. They do not work that far from home, but traffic congestion does not allow getting there faster; almost every day, they get stuck in traffic after dropping the kids at school. Although located far from home, the school is still easily reachable by bike, but bicycling is prohibited; it is too dangerous, considering the traffic flow in the area. So the children do not exercise much, either at school—where physical education has been removed from the curriculum—or at home, where they spend most of their time playing video games or watching television. They each have their own TV set and computer. They are now too old to play in the back yard, and there is no park at a walking distance. They cannot go anywhere on their own. Even their friends live too far to be visited without making prior arrangements, and they must be driven there by their parents. They live in such a huge house, with access to the external world through television and the Internet, that there is really no need to take the risk of going outside.

Tim and Laura eat at school, where their parents do not have much control over the type of food available. Last year, craving funding, the school signed an exclusivity contract with a soft-drink company, so the children are now fighting with their parents to be able to drink what they want at mealtime; their milk consumption has decreased considerably. They have gained weight too. Brian himself has a weight surplus, but he considers it normal because of his demanding sedentary work and his reluctance to do any physical activity after work; with his long commute, he has little time or energy to do so—he is exhausted from doing nothing physically! In any case, his backaches and joint problems prevent him from exercising. At thirty-eight, he believes it is too late to change his lifestyle. Tracy, who is forty-five pounds overweight, is aware of the problems induced by inactivity, although she does not know exactly why they have become so sedentary since they moved here. She became more concerned since she was diagnosed with diabetes last year. However, she does not exercise either, and she now suffers from a tennis elbow from her strenuous computer work. After trying many diet plans for years without success, she recently made an appointment for liposuction to restore her previous appearance, and Brian is considering doing the same. Thanks to plastic surgery, they will be able to go back to normal! And since they have good—although rather expensive—health insurance, doctors will take care of their health problems. After all, don't they have a great way of life?

Part 4

The Solutions

20
On Your Feet

I have two doctors, my left leg and my right.
—George Macauley Trevelyan

Why promote walking as a mode of transportation, rather than just recreational walking? Why not rely mainly on sports or other activities to remedy our sedentary lifestyle? The answer becomes evident only after looking at the causes of this lifestyle: utilitarian walking can act as a multipurpose tool. It can help prevent diseases and restore health; reduce traffic accidents, air pollution, and global warming; enhance road safety, a sense of community, and social equity; protect wildlife habitat, nonrenewable resources, and farmland; and, not least, save money, reducing the cost of health care, sewer infrastructure, cars, and gas; of building and repairing highways, roads, and parking lots; of time lost in traffic; and so on. It may not have a huge impact on any one aspect of life in particular, but its many small impacts would add up to substantial benefits.

Walking as a mode of transportation can be beneficial to anyone, whether they walk for recreation or exercise, and whether they drive or not, because it does not require any specialized equipment, and because it allows reaching a destination without any cost, provided it is not too far. Walking is a very democratic activity: it can be performed by the young, the old, the poor, the athlete, or the nonfit. Even sedentary people, those who do not want to get involved in any sport or competitive activity—they are many, and there will always be some—can enjoy walking.

A LONG SUMMER WALK

During the summer of 2003, Ariel Hames, a Harvard student, traveled twenty-three miles a day along the coast from Boston to New Brunswick, Canada, just to exercise and broaden her horizons by meeting new people (see wiscassetnewspaper.maine.com/2003-07-31/Canada_or_bust.html).

What about taking a three-mile walk every day for the same reasons?

Because it may reduce the level of traffic (just think about those 123 million daily trips under one mile), utilitarian walking can benefit motor-vehicle drivers too, since they would be less numerous on the roads; and it could help reduce traffic air-pollution by limiting the amount of unnecessary driving. It could also decrease the risk of road accidents and injuries because of lower traffic exposure.

Increased walking activity would improve public health and thus contribute to reducing escalating health-care costs. It would increase the fitness level of the population, helping maintain weight and even decreasing over-weight, making it profitable for taxpayers, who all share the burden of the health-care costs related to physical inactivity.

Utilitarian walking may also help develop a sense of community by providing more opportunities for informal social contacts and making neighborhoods safer because there are more pedestrians around, and more witnesses to watch what is going on. In a walkable environment, neighbors get to know and trust one another. An area devoid of pedestrians easily becomes a dangerous place where any kind of misbehavior is more likely to occur due to the absence of social pressure created by the presence of others. Encouraging people to walk will be a crime deterrent. Not do only people become healthier if they walk, but their neighborhoods become healthier as well, friendlier and safer. Children can play outside without direct supervision of their parents, and therefore be more physically active. The 1995 Oregon Bicycle and Pedestrian Plan noted that the number of people who walk (or ride bicycles) is an important measure of the quality of life of a community.

Most importantly, restoring the walkability of the urban environment is more likely to induce walking among people who otherwise would not be reachable by any campaign promoting increased physical activity. From the first steps of a child, walking is a step toward greater autonomy, and this is especially true for the elderly—those who are too old to drive or suffer from vision impairment or other physical disabilities.

There is no single solution for increasing walking activity. But the fact that it has been altered mainly by our lifestyle and environment should help point out the main avenues to follow.

Until now, solutions to the lack of physical activity have relied on individual behavior change, as for obesity. However, experience has shown that the fitness boom—organized sports and fitness programs—of the last decades was not enough to keep the whole population in shape. Most of us are not sufficiently motivated. And those who are not highly motivated are generally those who need it most. Daily, routine physical activity has almost disappeared due to a shift in the type of work, and to an environment unfavorable to nonmotorized transportation. Leisure time has been filled with sedentary activities such as television viewing and computer use. Physical inactivity is instilled very early in life, because parents believe it is too dangerous to let children play outside or go places on their own, due to the high level of traffic and to unfriendly neighborhood design that makes it potentially unsafe.

It would be surprising if a reversal of these trends could be brought about by relying only on individual willpower. Structural changes that enable the adoption of healthier lifestyles in our daily routine also need to be made. The relative failure of dieting solutions for obesity should be a good lesson for a successful battle against physical inactivity. On the other hand, societal strategies have proved very helpful in the fight against obesity.

WILLING TO WALK

Many signs indicate people are willing to adopt nonmotorized modes of transportation. A poll ordered by the Surface Transportation Policy Project in October 2002 that involved a national random sample of adults found that most Americans would like to walk more, but are held back by poorly designed communities that encourage speeding on the roads and dangerous intersections, and whose design makes it inconvenient to walk to shops and restaurants because the distances are too great. The main reasons Americans reported not walking were that "things are too far to get to" (61 percent) and that they "do not have enough time" (57 percent). More than half of Americans say they would like to walk more throughout the day rather than drive, either for exercise or to get to specific places. The most popular policies to encourage walking focus on reducing speeding—tougher enforcement of the speed limit, and designing streets with more sidewalks and safe crossings to reduce speeding. A majority favors making it easier for children to walk to school, improving public transportation, and increasing federal spending on pedestrian safety.[1]

Two surveys reported by the National Bicycling and Walking Study in 1992 examined the distance people were willing to walk for their utilitarian trips. Forty percent of Seattle residents considered the maximum distance suitable for walking on errands to be one mile or less, and 70 percent said two miles or less; overall, the people surveyed said they would consider a maximum walking distance of 2.1 miles.[2] In Canada, Ontarians said they would be willing to walk on errands or to work for about twenty minutes, which translates to about 1.25 miles.[3]

According to the Pedestrian and Bicycle Information Center, there is a growing demand for safe walking and bicycling facilities all across the United States.[4] The center, established in 1999 as a national clearinghouse on walking and bicycling for the U.S. Department of Transportation, provides technical assistance to help communities improve their quality of life through initiatives to increase safe walking and bicycling as a means of transportation and physical activity.[5]

In Canada, a national survey conducted in 1998 also indicated that people would like to walk or bike more if there were more suitable facilities; 80 percent said they would like to walk more frequently.[6]

WALKABLE CITIES

What a better proof of the willingness to do more walking than the popularity of walkable destinations for vacations? I mean not only hiking trips in the national parks, which are without any doubt a favorite, but also, and even more popular, visits to walkable American cities or small towns, and they are many. I had the chance to visit a few of them in many states—Alexandria and Georgetown, near Washington, D.C.; Bethesda, Maryland; Bar Harbor, Camden, and Kennebunkport, Maine; Petoskey, Charlevoix, Traverse City, and Mackinaw Island, Michigan; San Francisco, California; Ithaca, New York; Middlebury, Stowe, and Montpelier, Vermont; North Conway and Hanover, New Hampshire; Boston, Massachusetts; and many others. These are places cherished by pedestrians, places you feel safe walking even in the evening. They are attractive places, not only due to their historic character, but also because they rely on a model of development we crave, a walkable community where destinations can be reached on foot, where walking on pedestrian-friendly streets is a pleasant experience because architecture and

THE TEN BEST WALKING CITIES

Stating that walking is one of the best ways to stay fit, the American Podiatric Medical Association surveyed the ten best walking cities among the most populated ones, based on their pedestrian-friendly characteristics, such as the number of parks, the proportion of people walking to work daily, the crime rate, the pedestrian danger index, safe air quality, precipitation, the availability of podiatrists, health clubs, and sports stores, and the presence of a walking coordinator to develop special programs and encourage more walking within the city. According to these criteria, the best walking city was New York, followed by San Francisco, Boston, Philadelphia, Seattle, Denver, Washington, D.C., Chicago, Portland, and Cleveland (see www.apma.org).

even small things like street signs are nicely designed, where you can get some refreshment while you are walking around, where you can window shop instead of driving by a huge warehouse, a place where you feel at home—not your present home, but the one your parents or grandparents owned a few decades ago. There are thousands of places like these in the United States, and people just love being there. Most of these places are old towns, and we may think we visit them mainly for their historic character, although I suspect we also visit them because they are beautifully designed and illustrate the kind of development we favor, a human-scale development. The walkability of these cities attracts tourists and generates more income for their residents.

A short list of walkable communities across America was set up by Dan Burden, director of Walkable Communities Inc., but it can surely be added to and publicized to promote these communities' characteristics and help people who want to design pedestrian-friendly neighborhoods (see www.walkable.org). A more exhaustive list could be advertised at the state and federal levels, encouraging people to visit these cities. They do not have to be old or small; whether a city's growth is horizontal or vertical, its walkability can be improved or preserved.

In Canada, the city of Vancouver has achieved a high degree of walkability even in the new high-rise downtown neighborhoods. Trees, shrubs, and flowers can be found in the most unexpected places, even where there is very little space between the buildings. Bicycling is also very common. The city

WALKING CALORIES

How many calories are burned during walking? The answer depends on many factors: the weather conditions (air temperature, winds, and altitude), the soil nature and slope, and the body weight, height, age, and speed of the walker. According to Wendy Bumgardner, "A 35-year-old active male 5 feet 10 inches tall and weighing 170 lbs walking at 5mph on concrete in 72 degrees F will burn about 10.2 calories per minute. If he walks for 1 hour, he will burn a total of 612 calories. A 55-year-old sedentary female 5 feet 7 inches tall and weighing 150 lbs walking at 3 mph would burn 4.3 calories per minute. A one-hour walk would burn 258 calories."

One pound of fat equals 3,500 calories. So, to lose one pound, you have to cut your caloric intake or increase your level of physical activity to equal 3,500 calories. To me, this amount represents nearly six hours panting and sweating on my stationary bike!

Wendy Bumgardner provides her readers with a table illustrating the amount of calories burned per mile according to one's weight and speed. Her Web site (walking.about.com) also has a walking calorie calculator. Many pedometers now give the count of calories burned in addition to number of steps taken and distance traveled.

is renowned for its numerous parks, big and small; walking there gives the overwhelming impression that nature and urban development can cohabit harmoniously. Despite the city's population of two million, you feel as though you are in a garden inhabited by high-rise buildings. Stuck between the mountains and the sea, Vancouver had no choice but to limit sprawl and opt for a more compact model of development. Nevertheless, local authorities were concerned about protecting the environment and the spectacular scenery offered by the location. They never built an extensive freeway system and avoided massive spending on new roads and bridges. Transportation policies favored the development of a good transit system, which was made possible by the high-density residential development. Despite its annual population growth rate of 2.6 percent, Vancouver has not given way to sprawl.[7] It is surely one of the most beautiful cities of North America, as I noticed on my last trip there in April 2003. No wonder Vancouver attracts so many people who want to live there, despite its rainy climate!

21
The Benefits of Walking

The sum of the whole is this: walk and be happy;
walk and be healthy. The best way to lengthen out our days is
to walk steadily and with a purpose.
—Charles Dickens

EVERYONE WINS

Walking benefits not only walkers but also—as strange as it seems—drivers as well, because when short trips are made on foot, there are fewer cars on the road and consequently less traffic congestion, so the time spent driving is shorter, and the risk of accident smaller for the residual drivers. Fewer cars on the roads also means less traffic air-pollution and thus fewer people suffering from respiratory problems. Increasing the number of short trips made on foot protects—at the same time and in two different ways—young children, the poor, and the elderly, because they are more vulnerable to respiratory diseases and are also more likely to walk than any other age groups. Less traffic pollution means fewer respiratory problems among them, and less traffic decreases the risk of being hit by a motor vehicle for these pedestrians. It also improves their mobility and autonomy, decreasing their social exclusion and the burden associated with their dependence on other people. Opting to walk instead of drive, when the environment and distances make it possible, is a step toward a more equitable society.

A SAFER NEIGHBORHOOD

Walking makes an environment safer, as there are more witnesses around—more "eyes on the streets," in Jane Jacobs's phrase—more people you can

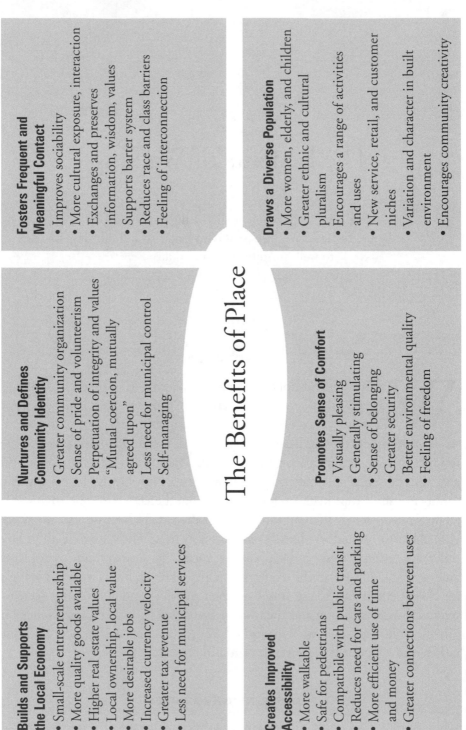

The Benefits of Place

Fosters Frequent and Meaningful Contact
- Improves sociability
- More cultural exposure, interaction
- Exchanges and preserves information, wisdom, values
- Supports barter system
- Reduces race and class barriers
- Feeling of interconnection

Draws a Diverse Population
- More women, elderly, and children
- Greater ethnic and cultural pluralism
- Encourages a range of activities and uses
- New service, retail, and customer niches
- Variation and character in built environment
- Encourages community creativity

Nurtures and Defines Community Identity
- Greater community organization
- Sense of pride and volunteerism
- Perpetuation of integrity and values
- "Mutual coercion, mutually agreed upon"
- Less need for municipal control
- Self-managing

Promotes Sense of Comfort
- Visually pleasing
- Generally stimulating
- Sense of belonging
- Greater security
- Better environmental quality
- Feeling of freedom

Builds and Supports the Local Economy
- Small-scale entrepreneurship
- More quality goods available
- Higher real estate values
- Local ownership, local value
- More desirable jobs
- Increased currency velocity
- Greater tax revenue
- Less need for municipal services

Creates Improved Accessibility
- More walkable
- Safe for pedestrians
- Compatible with public transit
- Reduces need for cars and parking
- More efficient use of time and money
- Greater connections between uses

Project for Public Spaces, 2005

connect with if something dangerous happens. A neighborhood constantly filled with pedestrians is under natural surveillance. The presence of familiar strangers is not only reassuring but can also bring more security to the residents of an area. Usually, you trust people you encounter on a regular basis more than you trust complete strangers. Walking in the course of daily routine increases the probability of meeting the same people over and over again, and of developing connections with them. It provides more opportunities for social interaction.

Aggression is more frequent in a deserted environment than in a place filled with people from different backgrounds. This explains why underground parking lots are excellent places for violence, as shown in the movies. Empty streets are much more dangerous than streets where pedestrians are constantly walking by.

By decreasing the level of unnecessary motor-vehicle traffic, walking makes the road safer. More pedestrians in an area forces drivers to slow down and be more careful. Pedestrians benefit not only from slower traffic but from less traffic as well, since shorter trips previously made by car can now be done on foot. The risk of accidents for pedestrians has been found to decrease with increasing pedestrian flows.[1]

A CLEANER ENVIRONMENT

Fewer vehicles on the roads when short trips are made on foot instead means less fuel consumption, less road construction and repair, less space devoted to parking, and lower taxes required to sustain this type of development. More pollution results from the first minutes of a car trip, because a colder engine generates more pollutant emissions;[2] so if shorter trips by car were replaced by walking, the positive impact on air pollution would be greater than the reduction in driving distance. The amount of money required for increasing nonmotorized travel (money and land devoted to sidewalks, paths, and bike lanes) is considerably smaller than the expenditures resulting from its absence. The amount of land waste is also much smaller.

Automobiles and roads also contribute to water contamination, and the 260 million tires thrown out every year in North America constitute another serious environmental hazard.[3] Replacing short driving trips with pedestrian excursions would help reduce this waste of materials, as well as reducing the erosion of soil and the fragmentation of wildlife habitat from excessive paving.

HEALTH BENEFITS OF WALKING

Even a moderate increase in walking (at least thirty minutes per day) can translate into health gains. Walking can:

- Improve fitness level
- Help control weight
- Reduce blood pressure
- Reduce blood cholesterol
- Reduce abdominal fat
- Protect against osteoarthritis and hip fracture
- Help develop and maintain muscle strength
- Help manage diabetes
- Increase aerobic capacity
- Protect against cancer and cardiovascular disease
- Relieve the symptoms of stress and depression
- Provide a higher degree of autonomy later in life

LESS TRAFFIC CONGESTION

Many drivers would probably show great interest if they were told there is a shorter way to get to their destination without getting stuck in traffic. This solution is available, but it requires a new transportation philosophy and some incentives. Even despite sprawl developments, where destinations are often too far to be reached on foot, more than one quarter of daily trips in the United States are still one mile or less, and half are three miles or less. That means almost half of car trips are superfluous and suggests a great opportunity for nonmotorized alternatives, and, consequently, fewer cars on the road. The adoption of walking and bicycling for shorter trips is not an altruistic behavior, since most people will benefit from it at some times.

A BOOSTER OF LOCAL ECONOMY

Pedestrian-friendly environments have been found to attract not only residents but also tourism. Their popularity indicates how much they are valued by consumers. Worries about a decrease in business if people cannot drive to stores and restaurants and parks nearby are not justified. In fact, the opposite is more likely to happen. An area with light traffic, or even completely devoid of motor vehicles, will attract more people, because it will be seen as more attractive, more livable, and safer. Window shopping, which is particularly good for small businesses, can bring in more customers than car driving. Car driving is slowly killing small businesses because it favors big-box stores. Some adjustments, like a delivery service for large orders, might be useful, especially for food stores.

HEALTH BENEFITS

The health benefits gained from increased physical activity—even if they are moderate or intermittent—are numerous and depend on the initial activity level. Sedentary individuals tend to benefit most from increasing their activity to the recommended level,[4] which makes this a particularly suitable intervention to be carried out among the whole population.

INCREASE IN FITNESS LEVEL. Regular physical activity helps develop and maintain higher levels of physical fitness. It plays a significant role in weight control, and it has also been related to a reduction in the occurrence of many diseases. Moreover, its side effects are minimal, compared to more vigorous physical activities such as sports. Jeremy Morris and Adrianne Hardman, two British researchers involved in health promotion and physical education, reviewed the health benefits of walking and noted that "low levels of walking are a major factor in today's widespread waste of the potential for health and well-being that is due to physical inactivity." Walking, they insist, "is a year-round, readily repeatable, self-reinforcing, habit-forming activity and the main option for increasing physical activity in sedentary populations."[5]

LOWER BLOOD PRESSURE. Walking reduces both systolic and diastolic blood pressure in adults, independent of changes in body composition.[6] It has been used successfully as a nonpharmacological method for treating people suffering from mild hypertension.[7] It has a beneficial effect on blood clotting, reducing the occurrence of stroke and heart disease.

CHOLESTEROL CONTROL. Regular exercise reduces the level of bad cholesterol (low-density lipoprotein) while increasing good cholesterol (high-density lipoprotein), providing better protection against atherosclerosis and coronary thrombosis.

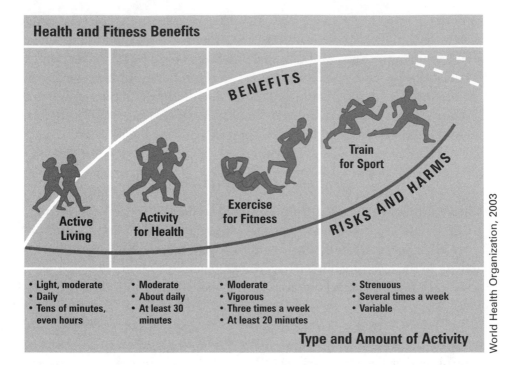

Health and Fitness Benefits

BENEFITS

Train for Sport

Exercise for Fitness

RISKS AND HARMS

Active Living

Activity for Health

- Light, moderate
- Daily
- Tens of minutes, even hours

- Moderate
- About daily
- At least 30 minutes

- Moderate
- Vigorous
- Three times a week
- At least 20 minutes

- Strenuous
- Several times a week
- Variable

Type and Amount of Activity

World Health Organization, 2003

LESS ABDOMINAL FAT. Exercise reduces the amount of abdominal fat.[8] In one study, even a low amount of exercise of moderate intensity led to a reduction of abdominal fat and global weight loss in nondieting overweight men and women; the minimum level for losing weight was as little as six miles per week of walking or other equivalent caloric expenditure.[9]

WEIGHT LOSS. A modest amount of exercise can prevent weight gain with no changes in diet, while more exercise may lead to important weight loss in initially overweight individuals.[10] A moderate-to-vigorous exercise program for previously sedentary and overweight women in combination with a decrease in energy intake resulted in 8 to 10 percent weight loss over a twelve-month period, higher levels of exercise being associated with greater weight loss.[11] After exercising, the metabolic rate remains high, increasing the level of energy expenditure well beyond the period devoted to physical activity. The failure of weight-loss programs until now may be due to the emphasis put on dieting without considering the potential benefits of exercise.

LOWER RISK OF CARDIOVASCULAR DISEASE. The cardiovascular benefits of walking are well illustrated by the results of a study of nearly 75,000 postmenopausal women who were followed for about six years. Those who walked regularly or exercised vigorously had fewer coronary events and fewer total cardiovascular events during the period; this was true for normal-weight, overweight, and obese subjects. Women who either walked or exercised vigorously at least 2.5 hours per week had a risk reduction of around 30 percent. Walking pace was important: walking at less than two miles per hour did not provide any risk reduction, and walking at more than four miles per hour led to a greater benefit than walking at two to three miles per hour. On the other hand, time spent sitting increased the risk of cardiovascular disease.[12] Walking plays a role in cardiac rehabilitation programs, as it can help reduce the risk of heart attack.

MENTAL HEALTH IMPROVEMENT. Physical activity raises tolerance to stress, improves the symptoms of anxiety and depression among people suffering from mild to moderate symptoms, and enhances psychological well-being, probably via the release of endorphins. Psychological improvements have been observed independent of changes in fitness.[13–15] Moreover, if walking is done in a social context, it increases the opportunity for social interaction, thus preventing isolation. It may also enhance the community sense and contribute to a decrease in fear of strangers.

THE AMISH AS AN EXPERIMENTAL COMMUNITY

The health benefits of physical activity associated with lifestyle are particularly noticeable when looking at groups such as the Amish community, whose members still refrain from driving automobiles, using electrical appliances, and employing other modern conveniences. Labor-intensive farming and walking for transportation seem to have limited weight increase among these people, despite a diet rich in fat and sugar. A survey carried out in an Amish community of southern Ontario involved anthropometric measures and the wearing of pedometers during a one-week period. The average number of steps per day reached 18,425 for men and 14,196 for women, well above the 10,000 steps recommended for a high activity level. One quarter of men and women were overweight, but obesity was nonexistent among men and was found in only 9 percent of women, probably due to their high level of activity.[16]

The Health Benefits of Place

Physical Activity

- Walkable—more likely to walk and more likely to walk longer distances
- Bikeable
- Recreation areas are better used
- Residents are more excited to get out of bed in the morning!

Consumer Benefits

- Closer connections between consumers and the products and services they purchase allows for greater education in the buying process and better access to the products and services they need to stay healthy (fresh nutritious food, drugs and health care, counseling, support groups, recreational activities, education centers, etc.)

Psychological Health

- Greater feeling of connection to one's surroundings
- Greater feeling of connection to the rest of the world
- Acceptance of differences
- Security to connect with others
- Visually pleasant yet stimulating environment

Social/Community Health

- People watch out for one another
- Teenagers and elderly are made to feel a part of the community
- There are things to do

Access to Health Products and Services

- Health services are more accessible and can be reached by public transit
- Local, fresh, nutritious food more available
- Better-quality water with centralized distribution and treatment
- Health information easier to dispense
- Access to health clubs and parks

Safety

- Fewer accidents (vehicle, bicycle, pedestrian, etc.)
- Fewer violent crimes ("eyes on the street")
- Less vehicle pollution
- Better able to organize against polluting organizations
- Health hazards are more eaasily discovered and dealt with

Project for Public Spaces, 2005

PROTECTION AGAINST OSTEOPOROSIS AND HIP FRACTURE. In the United States, 1.5 million fractures are attributed each year to osteoporosis. Physical activity increases bone density, thus providing protection against osteoporosis. Walking was found to protect against hip fracture among 61,200 postmenopausal women followed for twelve years.[17] These women did not suffer from osteoporosis at the beginning of the study. Walking for four hours per week or more was associated with a 41 percent lower risk of hip fracture among them. Even women at lower risk for hip fracture because they had a heavier cushioning layer of fat experienced a further reduction with higher levels of activity. Walking was found related to functional status fourteen years later in postmenopausal women, suggesting its importance in maintaining functional ability later in life.[18]

BETTER MUSCLE STRENGTH AND FLEXIBILITY. Walking helps develop and maintain adequate muscle strength for an independent lifestyle as we age. Improving balance, flexibility, coordination, and agility may also protect against falls among the elderly. Because it does not require strenuous efforts, walking rarely causes injury. Unlike in jogging, one foot is always in contact with the ground, which minimizes strain on feet and joints, thus decreasing the risk of injury. Walking may play a major role in the rehabilitation of elderly patients, for whom it is the most natural way of breaking the spiral of physical deterioration.[19]

INDEPENDENCE IN THE ELDERLY. One of the best illustrations of the autonomy of older pedestrians for me was a seventy-year-old Belgian man. On a visit with a friend to the city of Gant, we were sightseeing on foot, and he was walking behind us. In fact, he did not stay behind for long, because he walked much faster than we did. Reaching us, he saw we were tourists and offered to be our walking guide in the historic part of this old city. We had to increase our walking pace to follow him while he was telling us about the famous visitors of past centuries in his home town. He told us he was a member of a walking club that went hiking for days in the mountains. I was a little ashamed, realizing he was in better shape than people more than thirty years younger. The ability to walk does not decline with age, unlike with many sports.

REDUCTION IN DIABETES RISK. Because physical activity such as walking improves glucose tolerance and increases insulin sensitivity throughout the body, it helps reduce type 2 diabetes, a disease strongly related to sedentary lifestyle. Regular walking has even been associated with lower mortality among nearly 3,000 U.S. adults with diabetes in a study that followed them for eight years. The mortality rates were lowest among those who walked three to four hours per week. The authors concluded that one death per year may be preventable for every sixty-one people who could be persuaded to walk at least two hours per week.[20]

RELIEF OF CONSTIPATION. Walking may help relieve constipation, another adverse effect of our sedentary lifestyle. In the United States, this problem accounts for more than 2.5 million physician visits every year. It is among the most frequent reasons for self-medication, and is particularly troublesome in the elderly. More than $500 million is spent annually on laxatives. Exercise activates colonic transit.[21]

PREVENTION OF ERECTILE DYSFUNCTION. Walking may help reduce erectile dysfunction among adult men better than changes in smoking habits, obesity status, or alcohol consumption, as shown in a follow-up study of more than 593 adult men from 1987 to 1997.[22]

BENEFITS FOR PREGNANT WOMEN. Brisk walking is also a good and safe exercise during pregnancy because of its low impact. During the postpartum period, it can help restore muscle tone and normalize body weight.

PROTECTION AGAINST CANCER. Physical activity seems to have a protective effect against the risk of developing colon and breast cancer.[23] A study following nearly 75,000 postmenopausal women for 4.7 years observed a reduction in the risk of breast cancer with recreational physical activity, even though it was not strenuous.[24] Just three hours of moderate cycling a week was linked to a 34 percent reduction in breast cancer risk in Germany.[25] Daily routine exercise in adulthood was also found related to a reduction in endometrial cancer risk by researchers of the Vanderbilt University Medical Center in Nashville, Tennessee.[26]

AEROBIC CAPACITY IMPROVEMENT. Exercise such as walking stimulates the metabolic rate, enabling the body to extract a higher intake of vitamins, minerals, and trace elements from food.[27] The lungs take in more oxygen to deliver it to muscles and tissue, thus contributing to maintaining aerobic capacity even in older age. Brisk walking (between three and four miles per hour) improves cardiac performance, reduces the heart rate, and increases fitness level, providing greater endurance.

REDUCED RISK OF DEMENTIA. The risk of cognitive impairment in older age is lower among people performing regular physical activity.[28] Walking may help protect against Alzheimer's disease and other forms of dementia, as shown in both sexes in 2004. Among men, those who walked less than 0.25 mile per day were almost twice as likely to develop Alzheimer's disease or another form of dementia as those who walked more than two miles a day.[29] Women walking at an easy pace for at least 1.5 hours a week experienced less cognitive decline during the following years, compared to women who walked less than forty minutes per week.[30]

LONGER LIFE. Walking and climbing stairs were found to increase longevity among adult men,[31] while bicycling to work was associated with a reduction of mortality in both men and women.[32] A lower mortality risk among physically active people during leisure time was found not only in the United States, but also among Dutch, Finnish, Japanese, Swedish, and British populations.[33]

22
Individual Solutions

Take a two-mile walk every morning before breakfast.
—*Harry Truman (advice on how to live to be eighty,*
on his eightieth birthday)

Although the promotion of walking in and of itself does not appear to be a very successful solution to the problem of physical inactivity if it relies only on individual willpower, and if no effort is exerted to design more walkable environments, some solutions are nevertheless noteworthy.

WALKING PRESCRIPTION

A visit to the family doctor usually ends up with a drug prescription. But if the health problem is the result of obesity or physical inactivity, there may be other options for treatment, options free of the side effects of pills, which encourage the patient to play a more active role in his or her recovery.

An individual but still neglected approach to promote walking—or other types of exercise to reduce obesity or at least maintain weight—is through medical advice given to the patient by the family doctor. Considering the wide range of adverse health consequences of overweight, obesity, and physical inactivity, and the special relationship between a patient and family physician, there is little doubt that this health professional should play an active role in the promotion of healthier diet and exercise habits. Clinicians have a direct and personal access to a huge proportion of high-risk individuals. As a respected source of advice, they can successfully help and encourage their patients to modify their lifestyle by offering behavioral strategies. Family physicians can motivate patients to comply with their recommendations and assess even minor health benefits such as lower blood pressure and cholesterol levels. However, many clinicians do not routinely assess overweight or obesity among their patients in the course of the office visit; moreover, advice about weight loss rarely includes exercise counseling.

Even a modest amount of physician counseling could have a substantial public-health impact, considering the large number of people visiting a primary care physician.[1] Counseling is more effective if the patient understands that a vigorous exercise program is not necessarily needed, but that small changes in lifestyle that increase physical activity would make a difference. It is not an easy task for the physician to tell a patient he or she is too fat. It has to be done in a diplomatic way if the physician wants to keep patients and make them understand the problem has more to do with health than with aesthetics.

A survey carried out in Canada revealed that only a small proportion of family physicians provided exercise counseling to their patients, although nearly four times more acknowledged they should do so.[2] There are many reasons for this situation. Very often, family physicians do not feel confident about counseling practices due to a lack of training. They also face a lack of time to do so. Moreover, many of them think their patients would not exercise even if they provided them with counseling. And it is not always prudent to tell a patient he or she is so fat that eating better and exercising more to lose weight and become more fit are imperative. If the physician hurts a patient's feelings, the patient may seek another physician. Evidence for the effectiveness of the "green prescription"—written exercise advice—is still inconclusive, but many experts believe it is more effective than verbal advice only. In the battle against overweight and physical inactivity, a call to action for clinicians was provided by the 2004 February edition of the *Archives of Internal Medicine*.[3] Better knowledge of the guidelines would help physicians deal with obesity and a sedentary lifestyle from a prevention perspective.

STAIR CLIMBING

There are many ways to reintegrate walking into the daily routine, but it must be kept in mind that walking is a much more pleasant experience when the environment is nicely organized. Just think about climbing the

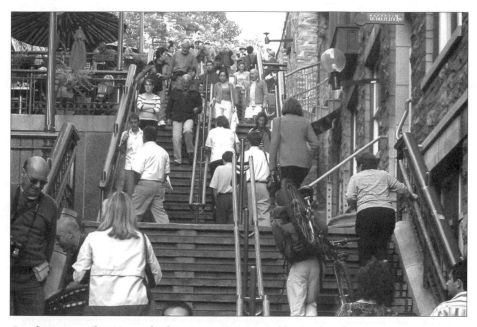

People are not reluctant to climb stairs. In some cities like Quebec, famous stairs are a tourist attraction. People even climb them with bikes on their shoulders, or carrying a stroller.

stairs at work. If your building is like mine, the stairs stand in the middle, where it is dark and gray—the color of concrete—and no one feels like exercising there, because it is too dull. My office is only on the fourth floor, and I rarely climb the stairs, because the environment is not appealing. If the walls were painted in attractive colors, more people would be likely to climb the stairs because it would be more inviting.

Very often, it is difficult to find the stairs in a building. Their location does not favor regular use, and the signs indicating where they are not always evident. They can be in a hidden corner where it may even seem hazardous to go. A person might even get stuck in a stairwell, because the door can be locked once they are inside.

Integrating the use of stairs in the daily routine is an easy, effective, inexpensive way to be more physically active. It can also save time at work, because waiting for the elevator often takes longer than taking the stairs. In his book on the fight against obesity, Kelly Brownell reviewed intervention studies aimed at increasing stair use, and all of them gave positive results.[4]

A significant increase in stair use was observed in an office building after an experiment in adding music and artwork to stairwells was carried out at the University of Minnesota.[5] Recently, the CDC decided to walk the talk, and took the initiative to improve the fitness level of its 9,000 employees in

Atlanta. It equipped the stairwells of its offices with music, new lights, and fresh paint to encourage workers to climb the stairs to exercise.[6] How can we expect people to exercise in a dull and dark place, where you can even get locked in? It is common sense that people would exercise more in an appealing environment. We try to integrate exercise into our daily life, but it usually has to be done in a dull and monotonous location. It is not very inviting to go out for a walk after dinner when you live in a house stuck between two highways, and where walking is possible only on a limited number of streets devoid of sidewalks.

Escalators also should be restricted. I was astonished on a visit to the San Diego Zoo in the early '80s when I saw an escalator going uphill outside. I could not imagine someone going to the zoo and not expecting to walk from one site to the next. Escalators cannot be used by people in wheelchairs, so most of those who use them are supposed to be able to walk. Unlike their European counterparts, Americans stop walking once they get on an escalator, which creates congestion. The only purpose of this perverse technology seems to be a reduction of human effort. Avoiding escalators when going to the shopping mall is a first step toward recovery.

Stair-climbing contests could be held in many office buildings, which would encourage employees to use the stairs daily to get fit enough to participate in the annual climbing marathon, in which everyone wins, in terms of health benefits. Stair use does not have to be restricted to fire drills; stairs should be used for exercise as well.

DOG WALKING

Dog walking seems another good opportunity to perform physical activity, since our pet companions have to go out for their basic needs and exercise. But people are inflicting their own sedentary lifestyle on their pets; many dogs now suffer from obesity because of lack of exercise and overeating. A study carried out in Australia found that more than half of dog owners did not walk their dogs;[7] nevertheless, on average, dog owners were found to walk eighteen minutes per week more than non–dog owners. Walking the dog was estimated to have a significant impact on direct health-care cost saving. About 40 percent of Australian households have a dog. In the United States, 36 percent of households own a dog; the statistics for lack of exercise are probably similar.

More and more cities across North America now have their annual "Mutt Strut," a special event where dog owners and their pets engage in a long walk to raise funds for some worthy causes; these events are often organized by the Humane Society. If your city does not already have an annual Mutt Strut, you might try starting one to raise money to fight diabetes, which is strongly linked to our sedentary lifestyle. This special event encourages dog owners and their companions to share precious exercise time together, as well as with other humans and animals, and increase public awareness of the importance of walking for health.

A study financed by Hill's Pet Nutrition, a pet food company, and performed by a team working under Dr. Robert Kushner, medical director of the Wellness Institute at Northwestern Memorial Hospital in Chicago, found that dog owners and their pets could lose weight and successfully stay

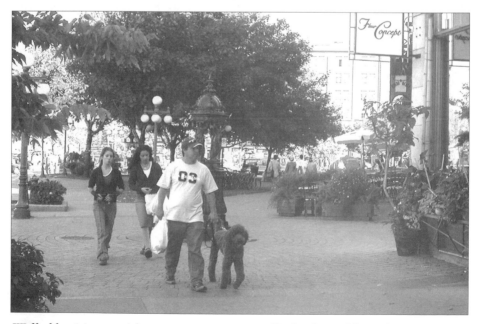

Walkable cities provide an opportunity to walk the dog safely and in a pleasant environment, which can benefit both the dog and the owner.

WALK-A-HOUND, LOSE-A-POUND

This program, implemented in the city of Lubbock, Texas, has been developed by the city's animal services department and health education team, and is open to anyone interested in getting a workout with a side order of animal interaction. It encourages people to register as walkers for the dogs in the city animal shelter, thus providing, as they say, "couch-potato humans and stir-crazy pooches with some much needed exercise." So far, about sixty people have signed up to walk dogs (see www.doh.wa.gov/cfh/steps/publications/walk_a_hound_packet.doc).

trim by joining a diet and exercise program together. Support from their beloved animals can give people the motivation to adopt healthier habits. This "people and pet weight management program" encourages dog owners to take daily walks with their companions, in addition to going on a low-calorie diet.[8]

However, even if you do not own a dog, or do not want to, some opportunities for dog walking are still available.

WALKING CLUBS

Many people do not walk in their neighborhoods only because they are alone. They may be afraid or lack motivation to do so. Or they may live in a place not suitable at all for pedestrians. A walking club membership could be a solution for them. The American Volkssport Association has a network of 350 clubs around the country and organizes more than 3,000 walking events each year. However, while this may help increase the physical activity and fitness level of those who participate, it does not improve the quality of the neighborhood itself.

STEP BY STEP . . . WITH A PEDOMETER

How many steps do we take during the course of a normal day? It is difficult to guess, because we walk countless short distances during an average day, from one room to another, from the desk to the printer, and so on. But do we walk enough to keep in shape, especially if we are sedentary? For most of us, these questions remain unanswered. But during the last few years, a small device designed to measure ambulatory activity in the form of step count—the pedometer—has become popular for assessing the level of physical activity and encouraging sedentary people to exercise more. Used at first on a small scale, it is now spreading to large groups of people— because it is simple and inexpensive—suggesting its appropriateness for public-health purpose.

America on the Move, a national walking program launched in July 2003 by Dr. James O. Hill, director of the Center for Human Nutrition at the University of Colorado in Denver, after a successful initiative he carried out in Colorado the preceding year, promotes the adoption of new behaviors to be more physically active and eat more healthfully to fight the obesity crisis and increase fitness. This initiative is dedicated to helping individuals and communities make positive changes to improve health and quality of life, encouraging stakeholders from the private and public sectors to be part of the solution by creating communities that support healthy lifestyles. It involves wearing a pedometer (step counter) to encourage walking 2,000 additional steps every day—the equivalent of a fifteen-to-twenty-minute walk. This small device acts as a motivational tool for exercising and is an easy way to measure your progress; clipped to the waist, it counts footsteps by detecting body motion and converts this into a distance on the basis of the length of the wearer's usual stride. Some models also calculate the amount of calories burned. The program also encourages people to cut out 100 calories a day from their food intake.

People usually walk about 5,000 steps a day; the recommended number of steps is 6,000 for health, and 10,000 for weight loss, which represents about five miles. This new gadget may not help everybody walk more, but it can make some people more conscious of how much they walk and give them quick and reliable feedback on their progress, in the same way a scale does for those who are watching their weight. Recent experiments have shown that setting daily step goals, keeping a log of steps walked, and wearing the pedometer all the time are linked to improvements in level of awareness and amount of physical activity, as well as fitness improvements such as increased energy, weight loss, and less illness.[9] Walking 10,000 steps a day or more was found effective in lowering blood pressure, increasing exercise capacity, and reducing sympathetic nerve activity in hypertensive patients.[10] By tallying the number of steps you take, the pedometer helps you appreciate how far you walk; it seems that people usually underestimate their walking distance.[11]

However, as the pedometer approach relies mainly on individual willpower and behavior, it would be more successful if it was reinforced by a reorganization of the built environment, to integrate walking into the daily routine by providing safe, convenient, and pleasant places to walk.

Dieting and fitness programs, which also rest on individual initiatives, have not always been successful in the long run. Nutrition specialist Marion Nestle of New York University has observed, "If recommendations to consume fewer calories have so little effect, in may be in part because such advice runs counter to the economic imperatives of our food system."[12] As she has reported, it is difficult to reduce the level of caloric intake when Americans are surrounded by 170,000 fast-food restaurants and three million soft-drink vending machines; no simple solution can be found in "an environment so antagonistic to healthful lifestyles." Or as noted by the authors of *Pedalling Health*: "Programs attempting to urge people to make healthy life decisions are doomed to failure if they are mounted within an environment that encourages unhealthy options."[13]

Changing the environment is often the key to a drastic change in behavior. It is what happened with smoking: restraining the number of places people were allowed to smoke made it a less convenient and less socially desirable habit. Changing the environment has an impact on social norms, which in turn have a strong effect on individual behavior. The best incentive for behavioral change is still the necessity provided by the environment. This perspective is relatively new, as can be seen in the 1996 Report of the Surgeon General on Physical Activity and Health, in which emphasis was still put on promoting physical activity via education and intervention programs for the individual or for groups.[14] Only a few pages dealt with environmental considerations. Nevertheless, the CDC recognized that the major barrier to physical activity is the model of development created by modern technology, car driving, and sprawl.[15]

23

Creating Walkable Environments

A city that outdistances man's walking powers is a trap for man.
—*Arnold Toynbee*

REVISITING ZONING LAWS AND POLICIES

Obsolete zoning laws have to be changed—or even abolished—to take into account the reality of the twenty-first century, in which residents do not need to avoid polluting industrial workplaces as they did fifty years ago. Since these laws were set up to protect citizens from air pollution and other deleterious conditions mostly linked to industrial plants by segregating living areas from workplaces, they should now be changed to favor a mixed-use environment for the same reasons. This new arrangement would reduce air pollution and accidents related to motor-vehicle driving, decrease inefficient land use, provide a safer environment, and supply opportunities for regular physical activity as part of the daily routine. Zoning laws were designed for a car-oriented environment and, in fact, inhibit the development of human-scale urban neighborhoods. In most places, zoning laws make it illegal or at least very difficult to build a smart community characterized by pedestrian-friendly streets and a compact mix of houses, workplaces, stores, and recreational amenities. Minimum parking requirements for stores and offices prevent compact development, thus increasing trip lengths, which encourages car travel at the expense of transit use, walking, or bicycling.[1] People are so used to zoning laws that they do not always realize their negative impact on their daily lives. However, some states are beginning to understand the value of mixed-use environments and are now promoting easier ways to go to work. The state of Maryland gave at least $3,000 to people to buy a home in areas closer to their places of work.[2]

As noted in the 2004 March edition of the *American Journal of Health Promotion*, zoning laws actually stand in the way of health-promoting community designs and are therefore not in the public interest.[3] People seem to forget that zoning is not immutable. In the past, it was used for public-health purposes, to prohibit stores selling pornography or prevent the construction of waste-disposal facilities.

REFOCUS URBAN DESIGN

Rebuilding cities and suburbs to make them pedestrian-friendly and to help fight physical inactivity and obesity is an overwhelming task at first sight. It seems to be an unrealistic solution for those who think that promotion of physical activity is the key to the problems created by a sedentary lifestyle, and that government intervention in citizens' lives should stay minimal. However, Rogan Kersh and James Morone, two professors of political science in Syracuse, New York, and Providence, Rhode Island, have shown how the American government has a long tradition of intervening in private behavior, from alcohol prohibition at the beginning of the twentieth century, to the current battle against smoking and illicit drugs.[4] Since the government is paying the price for the consequences of obesity and physical inactivity, its involvement in finding solutions to eradicate these problems is quite normal and even a sign of healthy concern, and it is a realistic step in the pursuit of efficiency. Not only does the tremendous impact of careless urban design not profit the country, but it can drive municipalities and the health-care system into bankruptcy and jeopardize the quality of the environment. The pro-sprawl movement—land developers, highway builders, and the petroleum industry lobby—may be too powerful to change our obesogenic environment without major public funding and policy reforms.

Fortunately, some groups, such as the Congress for the New Urbanism, with its new president, John Norquist—mayor of Milwaukee from 1988 to 2003, and the author of *The Wealth of Cities*—are working on solutions to repair the damage done to cities by sprawl during the last fifty years and rebuild more livable communities, revitalizing old downtowns and reestablishing more compact and walkable neighborhoods.

Nevertheless, even if we reverse the trend and go back to walkable en-

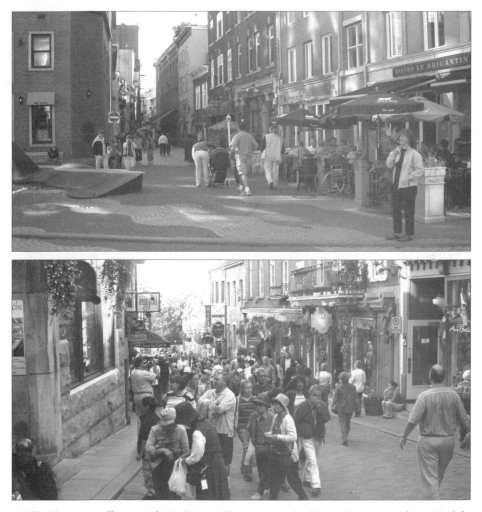

Walkable streets allow people with a stroller or in a wheelchair to enjoy outdoor city life; such streets benefit store owners too.

vironments, the change in behavior will not occur spontaneously. As Chuck Corbin, professor of exercise and wellness at Arizona State University in Tempe, has said, "You don't change habits in 15 minutes that have taken 50 years of bad behavior to establish."[5] It is not enough to make the destinations closer; people will have to relearn how to go places without a car. For their own good, they have to be reminded to burn calories instead of gasoline.

Even some minor adjustments can have beneficial effects: more and wider sidewalks, narrower streets, longer pedestrian lights, shorter blocks, turning radius of no more than fifteen degrees at the street corner, traffic-calming devices, planting trees along the streets for shade, more bike lanes, more bike racks and public benches, and restraining parking by de-paving parking lots or making them more expensive are among the easiest measures to encourage walking in the city.

Another alternative to restore a pedestrian-friendly environment, more commonly seen in Europe, involves closing certain streets to traffic for part of the day. Germany and Italy are two countries where the centers of many old towns and even bigger cities are closed to traffic for at least a part of the day, making it a more enjoyable and safer experience for pedestrians. Instead of pushing away visitors and jeopardizing the trade function of the area, these pedestrian streets attract more people because they create a more lively environment. It is common to see children playing in these streets as if the streets were part of their playground.

Europeans inhabit their streets much more than Americans do, and this fact has a tremendous impact on their social and political behavior. A good illustration is the reaction of Spanish citizens after the devastating multiple bombing of the trains in Madrid on March 11, 2004. More than eleven million people marched in the streets of Spain during the following days to defy terrorism, protest against it, and demonstrate in favor of democracy. The demonstration stressed the strong sense of solidarity among Spanish citizens, and marching together surely made them feel stronger and more powerful in the face of the invisible enemy. They rapidly understood the government's attempt to manipulate public opinion by attributing the at-tack to the Basque separatist movement, ETA, and they decided to overturn the government on election day, three days later.

In Canada, the city of Quebec stands midway between Europe and America in its urban design values. Since it was founded in 1608, its cen-ter was designed similarly to that of an old European town, with very nar-row streets, a compact mixed-use type of development, and stone walls surrounding it. Since the old part is built on a cliff, long stairways connect-ing the lower town to the center can be found all around. Along the streets, many cafés and restaurants have an open-air sidewalk section, and pedestri-ans are everywhere. Adjacent to this old part stands a huge park extending the pedestrian zone and overlooking the majestic St. Lawrence River from the top of the cliff, where the castle is located. In this area, pedestrians are kings. But outside the historic center, the city has suffered from sprawl, ex-cept for a few neighborhoods planned before the '50s, just as with other North American cities.

In the United States, Portland, Oregon, is probably the best example of what can be done at the municipal level to guide and regulate urban growth. Previously suffering from the same problems as other big cities, Portland initiated a vast reform as early as the '70s. Establishing a strong land-use policy, the city's leaders decided to contain sprawl and decrease traffic congestion by tracing a green border around the city, thus forcing a more compact model of development; they also implemented an efficient transit system based on buses and an urban light-rail line called MAX, and took measures to encourage nonmotorized travel. The "Skinny Streets" program recommended that new local streets in residential areas be only twenty feet wide, with parking on one side. All new buildings, including

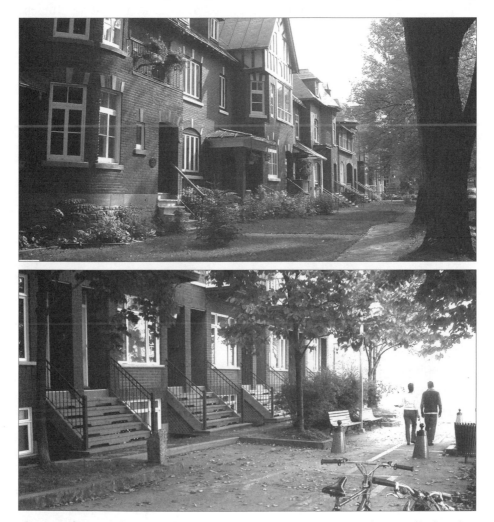

Compact housing does not always mean high-rise apartments, and it can be found in quiet neighborhoods.

167

garages, are people-friendly at street level, avoiding blank walls. Moreover, 1 percent of public construction funds is devoted to enhancing the physical attractiveness of the area through outdoor public art. Portland's parks system includes 200 green spaces. To prevent big-box stores from spreading all over the place, Portland now limits retail outlets to 60,000 square feet and restricts the number of parking spaces a new store may have to encourage the use of mass transit.[6]

Alternatives to car driving cannot succeed if there is no change in the type of development now prevailing. For instance, the low-density developments that characterize sprawl, along with its inherent segregation of functions, do not provide enough commuters to make mass transit an efficient mode of transportation. To solve this problem, transit-oriented neighborhoods are being developed, usually around a rail or bus station; stores where commuters can purchase what they need on their way home are located in a few commercial buildings. To justify frequent transit service, residential density cannot be too low. It is estimated that a transit-oriented development requires about seven residential units per acre.[7] Such neighborhoods typically have a diameter of one-quarter to one-half mile. By providing

TEN STEPS TO A WALKABLE COMMUNITY

Dan Burden, director of Walkable Communities, has identified the characteristics of walkable neighborhoods (see www.walkable.org/article 1.htm.):

1. Compact, lively town center
2. Many linkages to neighborhoods (including walkways, trails, and roadways)
3. Low speed limits on streets (twenty to twenty-five miles per hour in downtown and neighborhoods)
4. Neighborhood schools and parks
5. Public places packed with children, teenagers, older adults, and people with disabilities
6. Convenient, safe, and easy street crossings
7. Attractive and well-maintained public streets
8. Mutually beneficial land use and transportation
9. Celebrated public space and public life
10. Many people walking

transportation alternatives to car driving, this type of development reduces motor-vehicle ownership, travel, and expenditure. It also reduces paved land and traffic congestion, making such neighborhoods livable communities. People dependent on others for transportation in a car-oriented environment can use mass transit, which decreases the burden for those who usually have to drive them. The *Transportation Demand Management Encyclopedia*[8] and Oliver Gilham, in his book *The Limitless City*,[9] describe many case studies of such developments. For example, Arlington County, Virginia, has offered incentives to create mixed-use, pedestrian-oriented development surrounding transit stations, thus leading to greater use of mass transit to get to work.[10]

More compact developments are needed to increase transit use and walkability of a community. And it is possible to reach this goal even in already developed urban areas, especially in fighting urban decay. Here again, the city of Portland, Oregon, created original initiatives. Developers of the Buckman Heights Apartment project transformed a vacant inner-city auto dealership into a walkable and bikeable area with easy access to shops, work, recreation, and public transit.[11] In other places, parking lots have been converted into housing developments or recreational areas: around 200 units of affordable housing on an underused parking lot in San Jose, California, including space for play and work, as well as retail space accessible to residents and commuters; in Salt Lake City, a parking lot converted into a community center with an ice-skating rink, an amphitheater for concerts, and space for events and celebrations; in Racine, Wisconsin, a large parking lot and boat ramp replaced with a 3.5-acre waterfront green space connected to the city center. These Smart Growth initiatives reviewed by the Sierra Club have helped revitalize older city areas and make them more pedestrian-friendly.[12]

"Neotraditional" neighborhoods, promoted by the New Urbanism movement, share similar characteristics with transit-oriented developments, but they are usually located on greenfield sites, areas that have not previously been built upon. They are characterized by a higher-density, mixed-use environment, good street connectivity, and emphasis on other modes of travel such as walking and biking. In this type of development, culs-de-sac that restrain the free flow of pedestrians and traffic should be avoided as much as possible. To allow nonmotorized travel, the distance from the edge of the neighborhood to its center should be about one-quarter mile so it can be covered on foot in five minutes. This is exactly the distance between my house and the small shopping center at the end of my street. But to promote greater fitness, the distance could easily be doubled, and the walk would still be short enough to be comfortably covered on foot by a majority of people, even in the winter snow. The New Urbanism movement has created new communities of this type all around America and Canada.[13]

The Robert Wood Johnson Foundation in New Jersey is spending $70 million over five years on studies and programs to reintroduce walking as part of the daily routine in suburbs, cities, and towns.

In my own suburb, such a development was implemented about fifteen years ago. "The Campanile" was designed as a series of small commercial two-to-five-story brick buildings, with nice boutiques facing the street on the ground floors surmounted by condos and offices on the upper floors. The sidewalks are particularly wide. The architecture was borrowed from Italian towns, in which the center is marked by a bell tower, and from arcades, which protect pedestrians from rain, snow, or too much sun. In the center, a square is filled with public benches and a fountain, along with a few sidewalk cafés and restaurants, allowing people to take a rest, have a drink, or converse with each other. Fortunately, the area was already surrounded by trees. Around this small center, a relatively high-density type of development was favored consisting of four- or five-storied apartment buildings and condos. A little further, but still less than five minutes on foot, semidetached and single brick houses were built in what was previously an orchard. It is a place practical and safe enough to raise children or to attract retired people, so it is filled with residents of all ages; there is no high-speed traffic on the quiet streets of this neighborhood. Pedestrians are more numerous here than in other neighborhoods. A bus service every fifteen minutes connects this neighborhood with the other parts of the suburb and the center of the city. The success of this development has drawn more residents and inspired more construction, but efforts have been made to preserve the former landscape. Despite this success, there are still few places like this one.

TAME THE STREETS

In the past fifty years, streets have been designed almost exclusively for car circulation, as if cars were the only users. The streets are constructed to facilitate speed. However, this public space—for which everyone pays—is shared with many others: pedestrians, bicyclists, transit vehicles, trucks. Traffic engineers have forgotten that the role of streets goes beyond the purpose of circulation, and pedestrians have been ignored in the design of the

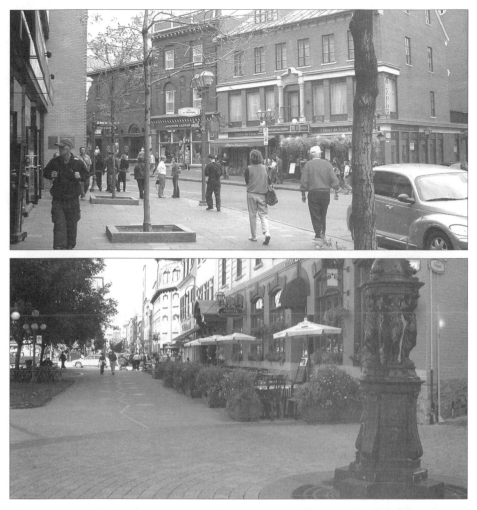

Mixed-use neighborhoods attract pedestrians and usually have high property values.

roadway system. As part of the human habitat, streets are the site of many social activities. Designing new streets or retrofitting the older ones should take this fact into account to increase their livability.

According to the authors of *Creating Walkable Communities*, "Streets are one of the most significant elements of our communities. How they are planned and designed generally determines how walkable the community or the neighborhood will be."[14] In a pedestrian-friendly environment, the street space must be safe and feel safe; it must also be comfortable and interesting, in the view of the New Urbanism movement.[15] People are not going to walk along streets with high-speed or high-volume traffic or that are flanked by plain walls and parked cars. Parking lots facing the street in front of buildings set too far back are not attractive to pedestrians either. Restraining parking space and moving it to the rear, or at least to the side, of buildings is among the possible solutions. Two-way streets are favored over one-way streets, because the latter encourage speeding. Narrow streets give a feeling of enclosure and comfort, especially when lined with rows of trees that not only provide shade but act as a buffer between pedestrians and the turbulence of the street. Narrow streets also help slow down the traffic flow. The recommended lane width is ten feet, which makes the streets easier for pedestrians to cross. The curb should be low enough to allow people to step on and off the sidewalk without any danger or discomfort. Most city streets in the United States these days have curb ramps that are flush with the street at crossing points so they can be negotiated by people in wheelchairs; this was required by the Americans with Disabilities Act of 1990.

Traditional street networks such as the grid pattern, which is characterized by a high degree of connectivity, is encouraged for nonmotorized use, because it reduces trip distance and increases the number of alternative routes, compared with the hierarchical pattern prevailing in the suburbs, with its low connectivity and its numerous cul-de-sac streets. Dead-end streets should be restricted to areas where there is no alternative due to the geography, because such streets impede easy travel from one area to another by increasing the walking distance between two points.

Promoters of neotraditional design favor parallel parking, which has been on the decline in most cities but is still very common in Europe and in older American cities such as Savannah, Charleston, Annapolis, Princeton, and Alexandria. Because it creates a bigger physical barrier between the street and the sidewalk, parallel parking helps protect pedestrians from moving traffic. It also eliminates the problem of bikers smashing into carelessly opened car doors. Parallel parking slows down traffic more than in-line parking and also gives more protection to the driver when getting in or out of the car. Moreover, it allows more parking spaces along the street than in-line parking.[16,17]

A new concept has recently been developed known as "naked streets," or streets without any markings, barriers, traffic signals, or traffic lights. This revolutionary idea was first suggested by Hans Monderman, a Dutch traffic engineer. Without street signals, drivers, cyclists, and pedestrians are forced to interact, make eye contact, and adapt to the traffic instead of relying blindly on external signs. Monderman says behavior is then negotiated through eye contact. According to him, when drivers stop looking at signs and start looking at other people, driving becomes safer, because instead of focusing on lights and other signals, they have to pay attention to what is happening around them and to adjust their driving accordingly.

It may sound dangerous and crazy at first, but the implementation of naked streets in a number of European communities has been very successful at reducing both traffic speed and accident rates. Urban planners in Holland, Germany, England, and Denmark who have experimented with this new approach to traffic management have found it safer than the traditional model based on heavy regulations. Among other benefits were a decrease in trip duration for drivers and a boost for businesses along the roadway. Even big cities like London are now trying it. You could argue that American cities and philosophy are different from those of Europe. But who would not like to feel safer when crossing the street, or get to destinations more rapidly without having to wait at red lights or stop signals?

REINTRODUCE SIDEWALKS

Reintroducing sidewalks into neighborhoods is probably one of the easiest way to increase their walkability, although by itself it would not be sufficient. The benefits of more sidewalks are double: first, they allow pedestrians to walk more, and more safely—which could be a major improvement for the mobility of children and the elderly, with a resulting reduction of the burden on those who have to drive them now; and second, sidewalks decrease the width of the streets, thus encouraging drivers to reduce their speed. Streets with pedestrians also make a neighborhood safer.

Confronted with the problems brought up by traffic congestion and obesity, many cities are now focusing on increasing their walkability as well as their public transit use. The Atlanta region is spending $175 million to build 385 miles of sidewalks by 2005. In Charlotte, $10 million has been allocated to build sidewalks in places that never had them; less than half of Charlotte's 2,800 miles of streets have sidewalks on one or both sides. The city of Oakland passed a pedestrian master plan to improve its already walking-friendly design; city officials want to make sure that people can walk to a new bus system. To reach this goal, they will upgrade sidewalks and intersections near transit stops. Other pedestrian improvements were recently made in the area of Rochester, New York, where many people walk; the region spent $5 million to upgrade walking and biking trails in 2002.[18]

But sidewalks cannot be effective if they are not specially designed to

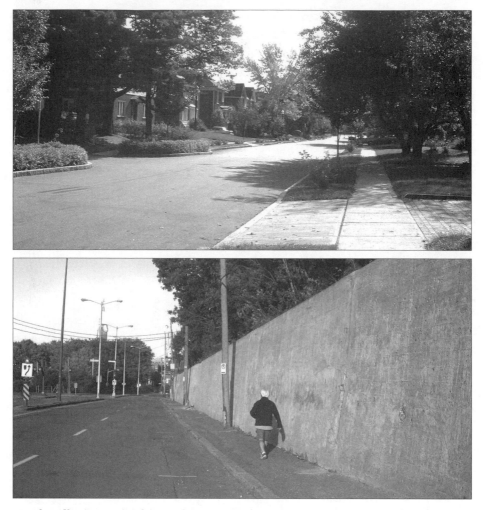

A sidewalk is not enough to make a street safe or pleasant. Here, the concept of "eyes on the street" developed by Jane Jacobs is particularly meaningful.

facilitate walking. Guidelines for the design of sidewalks have been illustrated for the Mid-America Regional Council, Kansas City, in a publication prepared by the Bicycle Federation of America in 1998 titled "Creating Walkable Communities: A Guide for Local Governments." They recommend sidewalks a minimum of five feet wide, with a minimum two-foot planting strip separating them from the street, and measures to limit the slopes giving access to garage driveways on residential streets, which are difficult for people—especially for the elderly and disabled—to negotiate when they are too steep. Sidewalks should be eight feet wide in business and commercial areas.

Building new sidewalks cannot be an effective measure, however, if there is no destination reachable on foot, or if there is not enough lighting. Sidewalks not only have to be available, they also need to be safe, convenient, and enjoyable to be used effectively. They should be free of objects limiting their walkability, such as utility poles, tree roots, advertising signs, and trash containers. A "Pedestrian Facilities Users Guide" was developed by the Federal Highway Administration in 2002.[19]

ADD BIKE TRAILS AND WALKING PATHS

Considering the high level of bicycle ownership, and the fact that half of daily trips in the United States are three miles or less, cycling could be a good opportunity to reduce traffic congestion and enhance the fitness level of the population, as well as the autonomy of groups such as children, the elderly, and people who cannot afford to buy a car. Cycling is affordable to almost anyone and does not require a source of energy other than human effort. But cycling as a mode of transport will not increase unless it is promoted. Among the proposals to make it safer and more convenient are to increase the cost of car use, clarify cyclists' legal rights, expand bicycling facilities, make all roads bikeable, hold special campaigns such as employer-based promotions, link cycling to wellness, and broaden and intensify political action.[20]

Road improvements should be made to allow safe bicycling. This could benefit up to 50 percent of the population living within five miles of work, a distance easily covered by bike.[21] Such measures, coupled with facilities such as bike racks and showers at work, could have a positive impact on the health of employees.

Three general categories of bikeways have been identified: bike paths (or trails) on rights-of-way separated from roadways; bike lanes on roadways separated from motor traffic by a barrier or a painted line; and bike routes on roads shared with cars or sidewalks shared with pedestrians.[22]

The availability of bike trails and walking paths induces people to use them simply because they are there, thus promoting physical activity, even among those who otherwise do not intend to exercise. In the mid-1960s, the "rail-to-trail" movement began converting abandoned or unused rail corridors into public trails, mainly for walking, inline skating, and biking, making it safe and pleasant to exercise or to reach destinations in a traffic-free environment. There are now around 100 million users for the 13,150 miles of rail-trails in most states nationwide.[23] Because of their predominantly rural location, these trails are used mainly for recreational cycling rather than for utilitarian trips. They do not necessarily connect with everyday destinations. On the other hand, the presence of high-voltage power lines over these pathways raises concern about potential adverse health effects resulting from exposure to electric and magnetic fields emanating from these lines.

In the United States, less than half of the municipal and country parks and recreation departments provided fitness trails, 29 percent provided hiking trails, and 21 percent provided bicycle trails.[24]

This kind of initiative is also spreading to other countries and suggests a strong potential for increasing bicycling as a mode of transportation or as a leisure activity. In eastern Canada, where I live, many defunct railroads are being transformed into bike trails, and they are now used by many people who were previously more sedentary because biking on the streets did not feel safe enough. Families and older citizens can frequently be seen riding along these trails. Since such trails cover very long distances, experienced cyclists can enjoy them too. In Australia, the New South Wales Road and Traffic Authority completed the construction of a ten-mile-long rail-trail cycleway in Sydney in 2000 as part of a Bike Plan to encourage alternative modes of transport and promote physical activity.[25]

Not everyone wants to separate biking routes from roads. Sometimes bike lanes are preferable to paths, especially when there are frequent intersections and private driveways along the way. In urban areas, creating bike paths might require redesigning the street network, whereas bike lanes could be implemented without any major changes.

At the federal level, some efforts have recently been made to help develop nonmotorized modes of transportation. Under the ISTEA's Enhancements Program, $972 million in federal funds was allocated for bicycling projects, and most of the expenditures were used for off-highway paths and trails. Only 13 percent went to on-road bicycling facilities. The Pedestrian and Cyclist Equity Act of 2003 (PACE) proposed to establish a $250 million Safe Routes to School five-year program to support the emerging movement, to fix roads near schools, and to encourage children to walk and bike to school. It also planned to establish a transportation and active-living program to integrate land-use and transportation planning to promote nonmotorized travel choices, incorporate pedestrian and bicycle-friendly features into community planning or legislative initiatives, enhance accessibility and mobility initiatives for the disabled, and implement communications and marketing strategies to promote physical activity.

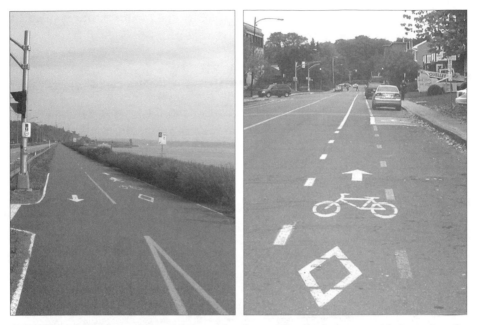

Bike lanes along the streets and bike paths along urban highways provide incentives for more cycling.

As part of a holistic approach to a walkable environment, the Philadelphia urban planner and author of *Design of Cities*, Edmund Bacon, developed the concept of the "greenway." The East Coast Greenway, the urban alternative to the Appalachian Trail, began in 1991 to establish a multimodal long-distance transportation corridor for cyclists, hikers, and other nonmotorized users connecting cities from Maine to Florida (see www.greenway.org). The greenway will enable residents to travel short distances from their homes to local points of interest, while contributing to reduced roadway congestion, improving air quality, assisting local economic development, making better connections among people and communities, and helping create new public space. The East Coast Greenway Alliance, a national nonprofit organization, provides the vision to make the linkages and the coordination to make it happen. Crossing the country from east to west, the American Discovery Trail, a nonmotorized recreational trail, stretches across more than 6,800 miles and fifteen states, linking communities, cities, parks, and wilderness areas.[26]

While hiking in the gorgeous scenery surrounding Sedona in Arizona a few years ago, I was stunned and annoyed to see and hear so many cars passing by, ruining the peacefulness of the area. I thought it would also be a very nice place for bicycling if there were not so much traffic. It is such a splendid area, equipped with so many recreational facilities, but spoiled by the overwhelming presence of cars!

CREATE PARKS INSTEAD OF PARKING LOTS

The lack of parks in the suburbs is probably due to the common belief that there is no need for them, since private houses are surrounded by large areas of lawn—not very useful, however, for children's activities such as biking and roller-blading. This belief does not take into account the difference between the functions of private and public spaces.

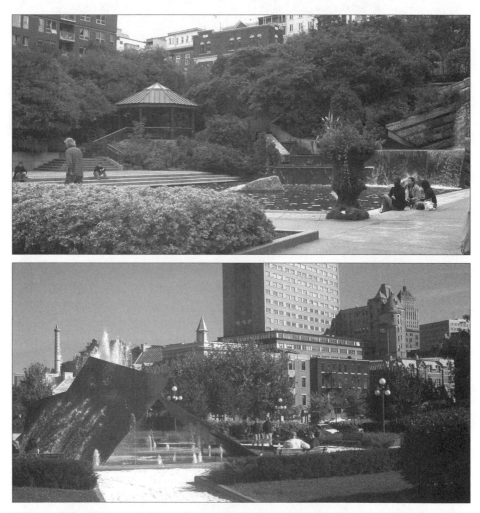

Urban parks give more value to the center of a city, providing spaces to rest and opportunities for social interaction.

Public parks are not just areas large enough to accommodate recreational activities. They are a significant part of the public realm, and in this respect, they provide gathering places for communication among people and supply the setting for organized or informal activities of all kinds. They do not have to be very large. In fact, the creation of small parks should be encouraged for two reasons: it is much simpler to create small parks in already developed areas, and supervision is also easier in smaller parks, making them safer places for children, as well as for adults. Even if they do not have trails or other recreational facilities, their proximity itself is a motive to exercise. Since they can be closer to home than larger parks, they encourage people to go there on foot instead of driving. In such places, pedestrians can stop along their way to rest for a while. These parks can be seen either as stopping places or as destinations, where someone can relax, read a book, walk the dog, watch other people passing by, or just take some fresh air. They should not be designed as if they were decorations, but as comfortable outer rooms. Small parks—or public squares—can improve the sense of community in a neighborhood. Whatever their size, they contribute to the livability of an area.

Greenways should allow pedestrians and bikers to travel from many parts of the city to its center, as well as to its outskirts. Long strip parks are particularly suitable for walking and bicycling and can be developed along waterfronts, where the natural scenery is one of their greatest assets. Unfortunately, many waterfronts have been invaded by roadways, depriving residents of the neighborhood of potentially splendid recreational areas. But in some places there has been a reversal. As part of a program to restore the livability of the urban community, an initiative of the mayor of Milwaukee, John Norquist, led to the demolition of the Park East Freeway, freeing up twenty-six acres of riverfront for smart-growth development, and the creation of the three-mile-long Riverwalk along the Milwaukee River.[27] In Tennessee, the city of Chattanooga cleaned up its seriously polluted river to create a riverfront park and a promenade, which now attract people and wildlife.[28] Zoning should protect the public and recreational potential of these areas by limiting their use for car circulation or upper-income residential projects; policies allowing the development of greenways and trails should also be encouraged.

Although an excellent location for recreational physical activities, large parks also help preserve open space and natural areas in or around cities. They attract not only residents but also tourists. Many big parks are famous nationwide, and even worldwide. They allow residents of cities to keep in touch with nature, especially those who cannot afford to get to the countryside or who cannot take the time to do so.

RESTORE PUBLIC SQUARES

Is there a free and attractive outer space within a mile that you can walk to, gather with other people, and sit? Probably not. Public squares, so common and cherished in European cities, have been forgotten in car-oriented developments. These places, usually located at the heart of a city, play an important role in social life, and their disappearance confirms the near-extinction of the public realm. When available, they can also motivate residents from an area to go for a walk. Public squares flourished in the early Spanish settlements of North and South America. The city of Sucre in Bolivia, designed with great taste in the seventeenth century, still has among the most beautiful squares I have seen in the world. Surrounded by astonishing architectural treasures, these squares are places where people can gather, sit down, read the newspaper, or listen to musicians. All this, despite the fact that the city is in one of the poorest countries of the Americas.

Squares do not require large pieces of land filled with tall trees. They can be located in small vacant spaces and have as focal point a statue, a sculpture, or a fountain. Because of their size, they are safer places, and they can be easily integrated in an already built environment. However, not all squares are

THE TWENTY-TWO SQUARES OF SAVANNAH

Savannah's legendary squares were designed in the eighteenth and nineteenth centuries as an integral part of the city's downtown. They are about 200 feet from north to south, and between 100 and 300 feet from east to west. All have attractive and convenient seating; many have fountains and monuments at their centers. Every day, thousands of tourists walk through or drive or ride around them. Visitors are stunned by their first experience in the squares. They have become Savannah's image in the minds of millions throughout the world. They are home to many cultural institutions and museums and the scenes of public celebrations. They are accessible and linked to their surroundings. Every year, the beauty and vitality of Savannah attracts 5.5 millions visitors (see www.pps.org).

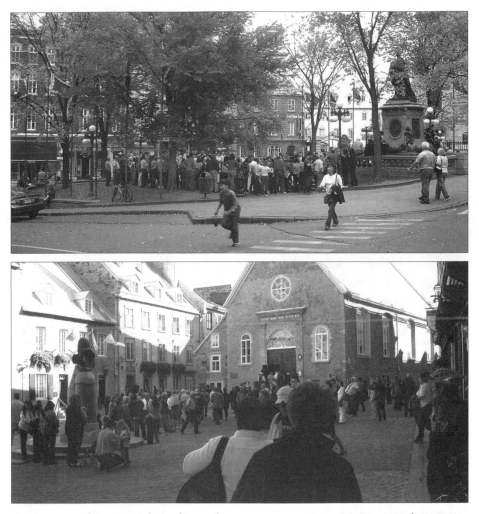

Squares are often great places for performance events. Here, musicians and magicians attract passers-by.

successful. In its evaluation of more than 1,000 public spaces around the world, Project for Public Spaces—a New York nonprofit organization helping people create and sustain public spaces that build communities—found that successful spaces share four qualities: they are accessible and comfortable places where people can socialize and engage in activities (see www.pps.org). In Germany, for example, some squares are gathering points for chess players. In addition to the usual tabletop chess boards, giant game boards are laid out on the ground; players walk around the board to move the huge pieces from square to square, while spectators watch in silence.

Project for Public Spaces has also identified the most common reasons why some public spaces fail. Among them are lack of places to sit, lack of gathering points, paths leading nowhere, blank walls, domination by vehicles, poor entrances, and visually inaccessible spaces. In other words, just putting benches along a blank wall in an empty area devoid of interest does not make it a public square.

At first sight, squares may seem to be an inefficient use of land in urban areas where land prices are very high. But such places have been found to support the local economy, attract tourism, and reduce crime, while improving the environment, pedestrian safety, and public health as well (see www.pps.org).

WALK TO SCHOOL

One of the best ways to make people walk as adults is to get them used to it as children. Specific programs such as Safe Routes to School encourage walking or biking to school using a comprehensive approach that includes design improvements such as crosswalks, expanded sidewalks, traffic calming, bike lanes and paths, public enforcement of traffic laws around schools, and education programs. They also fund local projects to improve road safety and children's mobility, health, and fitness, build stronger community ties, and reduce traffic congestion and air pollution. These programs involve parents, school teachers, community volunteers, and traffic engineers as well. They were reviewed nationwide in a report published by the Surface Transportation Policy Project in 2002.[29]

Walk to School Day is an initiative held in October every year. This event, which involved only two schools at its beginning in 1997, now has more than 2,800 participating schools in all fifty states, and more than three million walkers in twenty-nine countries worldwide, illustrating the awareness of walking benefits for children under safe conditions, and the potential for a major change in modes of transportation.[30] In California alone, the state has dedicated $20 to $25 million a year during the last three years for the Safe Routes to School program, contributing to sidewalk improvements, traffic calming, speed reduction, pedestrian- and bicycle-crossing improvements, on-street bicycle facilities, and traffic-diversion improvements, as reported by the STPP California 2003–2004 initiatives.[31] The beneficial impact of this program did not take long to manifest, as shown by a study carried out in Marin County, just north of San Francisco, funded by a grant from the National Highway Traffic Safety Administration. After two years, the fifteen participating schools reported a

64 percent increase in walking and a 114 percent increase in biking.[32]

The effectiveness of these programs will be limited if physical education is not reintroduced into the school curriculum, along with efforts to stop the overexposure to junk food, snacks, and soft drinks in the school cafeterias. Lack of money should never be an argument for restricting the availability of physical education, unless the emphasis is put only on competitive sports requiring specialized equipment. Physical education relying on games and walks costs almost nothing and does not emphasize performance, which can be extremely discouraging for those who are less talented. Jumping rope, for example, is not very expensive but can be good exercise for children in elementary school. In Vancouver, some teachers ask their students to jump in the classroom between lesson periods; this exercise is supposed to help reinforce the bones. Very early in life, children have to learn to stay still, which is against the principles of healthy development. The best way to learn is not necessarily to sit down all day.

PROMOTE TRANSPORTATION ALTERNATIVES

The good thing about public transit is that the idea can be sold for more than one excellent reason, so it has a better chance of rallying public opinion. Developing transportation alternatives to the car encourages people to walk more, thus reducing car driving and its impact on air pollution, traffic congestion, and road safety, while at the same time increasing the level of physical activity in the population. Public transit is closely linked to walking; if it is to be effective, most people should be able to reach the rail, tram, or bus station on foot. Policies favoring transit will therefore also encourage walking. The promotion of public transport and walking creates greater equity in transportation by allowing those who cannot drive to reach destinations at an affordable cost. The urban poor, older citizens, and children then gain a higher degree of autonomy, allowing them to rely less on car drivers.

The Intermodal Surface Transportation Efficiency Act (ISTEA) of 1991 and its successor in 1998, TEA-21 (the Transportation Equity Act for the Twenty-first Century), led to an innovative approach to transportation by allowing new strategies to address the problems encountered, and by taking into account questions such as social equity, economic efficiency, environmental protection, energy conservation, pedestrian and biker safety, and impact on quality of life and community livability.[33] Emphasizing public participation and a holistic approach to planning made possible diversification of spending on public transportation. The emphasis is now on choice. From there, it became possible to spend a significant amount of federal transportation funds on nonmotorized modes of travel, such as mass transit, walking, or biking. Between 1990 and 2001, the amount spent on these projects went from $7 million to $313 million. Nevertheless, of the $50 billion given to the state departments of transportation between 1992 and 1999, less than 7 percent went to alternative-choice projects. In Tucson, for example, more than 200 miles of on-street bike lanes were installed during this period. In Seattle, the 1,200 city buses were equipped with bike racks. But most states continue to spend the majority of federal transportation funds on highways. During the 1990s, transit funding was still less than funding for highways, although it increased by 75 percent. But a new federal transit program called New Starts is funding new rail and bus infrastructure and has allowed many cities to open new transit systems.[34]

Following this funding, many transit systems were developed during the '90s. The MetroLink light rail system in St. Louis opened in 1990 and was carrying 40,000 daily riders only two years later. In Dallas, the DART light-rail system opened in 1996 and now has forty-four miles of track supporting 60,000 daily commuters; the transit agency and the city are promoting transit-oriented development opportunities around the stations. In Denver, a light-rail system connects suburbs from all directions to downtown, and here too it has led to the development of transit-oriented communities. Salt Lake City's light-rail system, TRAX, opened at the end of the '90s and is now acting as a catalyst to revitalize the city's downtown; it has led to the creation of many transit-oriented neighborhoods all around the city.[35–37]

Other initiatives have led to the reinforcement of the bus network, which can be more efficient when there are designated bus lanes; otherwise they get stuck in traffic like cars. According to Jane Holtz Kay, bus and rail are complementary rather than competitive, and funding one should not be done at the expense of the other.[38]

An innovative way to promote transportation alternatives and thus decrease traffic congestion was implemented in London in February 2003 by Ken Livingstone, the city's mayor. To reduce traffic in the crowded eight-square-mile city center, a $9 traffic toll was introduced for every private car entering this part of the city on weekdays between 7:00 a.m. and 6:30 p.m. at one of the 174 designated entrance and exit points. Taxis, buses, electric cars, motorcycles, and emergency services vehicles are exempt from the charge. Those who try to avoid the toll are detected with the help of a sophisticated camera system and are fined about $130. For the purpose, 688 cameras were installed at 203 locations to record license plates. One year later, traffic has fallen by 20 percent, improving travel time by 5 percent. Before the anticongestion program, the average speed in the area was about nine miles per hour—three miles less than at the beginning of the twentieth century, when horses were the main form of transportation.[39] Road-traffic emissions and fossil fuel consumption have also been reduced. A majority of the reduced car trips were replaced by the use of public transportation. Over 40 percent of residents living within the charging zone said it has become a better place to live. England is also facing an obesity problem, and the mayor of London now wishes to increase pedestrian trips of two miles or less by 10 percent before 2015. Every day, 110,000 car drivers pay the toll and each month, 165,000 fines are given to offenders. The funds will be used to improve public transit.

One of the responsibilities of the mayor is to improve the health of Londoners, and the Greater London Authority obliges him to consider health, equality, and sustainability as themes underlying all his policies.[40] Improvements in the public transport system are also aimed at making London a more accessible city, enhancing its economic development, leading to more job creation, and addressing the problem of social exclusion. The transport strategy relied on a health-impact assessment with recommendations for improvements.

In the United States, incentives to use mass transit have taken other forms. For example, some employers pay monthly subsidies to their workers to ride public transit instead of commuting by car. A California statute requiring certain employers to allow their workers to receive a cash payment instead of parking subsidies was found to increase transit use by 50 percent and bicycling or walking to work by 39 percent.[41]

IMPLEMENT TRAFFIC-CALMING DEVICES

Many people wish the traffic flow were lower in their neighborhoods. They also dream about drivers adopting a slower pace, so children could be safer and the level of noise lower. Fortunately, there are other options than police surveillance to make this dream come true, such as modifying the built environment to increase the difficulty of driving fast in residential areas, or rerouting heavy traffic.

Traffic-calming devices were designed to reduce vehicle speed and volume to make possible friendly coexistence of motorized and nonmotorized travel and increase everyone's safety, thus encouraging the use of other modes of transportation such as walking and biking. These devices are also very effective at reducing the number and severity of crashes. Traffic calming was developed in Europe, where its use is very common. Some traffic-calming strategies have been used for a long time: speed limits, vehicle restrictions on particular roads, traffic circles, and median islands. Others, like speed bumps, raised crosswalks, diagonal diverters, curb extensions, chicanes, and chokers, are less common and may annoy drivers not used to them. Some devices require only minor changes to the streets, while others involve a complete redesign of the roads on which they are implemented. In Europe, for example, it was found that converting conventional intersections to roundabouts can reduce the rate of pedestrian accidents by about 75 percent.[42] In the United States, the Insurance Institute for Highway Safety in Arlington, Virginia, showed that converting stop signs and traffic-signal control to modern roundabouts at twenty-four intersections led to a 38 percent reduction in the severity of traffic accidents and a 76 percent reduction in injuries.[43]

According to the Local Government Commission Center for Livable Communities in Sacramento, California, reducing traffic noise, speed, and

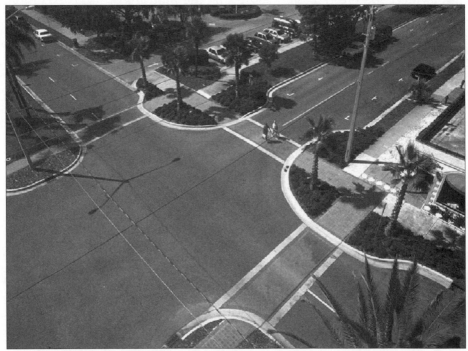

By decreasing the speed of traffic, diverters, speed bumps, and curb extensions can help restore a walkable environment.

air pollution by introducing traffic calming can increase property values because of the resulting better quality of life.[44] It is not rare to see traffic-calming devices on the streets in affluent neighborhoods. In his study of traffic-calming benefits, costs, and equity impacts, Todd Litman from the Victoria Transport Policy Institute in Canada reported that a five-to-ten-mile-per-hour reduction in traffic speeds increased adjacent residential property values by around 20 percent; traffic restraints reducing volumes on residential streets had the same effect, enhancing the livability of these areas.[45] Homebuyers are willing to pay more for a house in a pedestrian-friendly environment, especially when combined with land-use mix. Traffic calming has also been found to reduce the frequency of crashes and pedestrian injuries, improving the safety of the area. By facilitating nonmotorized transportation, traffic calming contributes to community interaction and simultaneously discourages antisocial behavior. It can also make an area more attractive.

The effect of traffic calming is expected to be greater in areas where walking and cycling are most likely to occur: residential neighborhoods, commercial centers, and schools and recreational centers. The impact is enhanced when other improvements such as sidewalks, bike paths, or public transit service are implemented at the same time.[46]

Traffic-calming experiences throughout the United States and Canada were reviewed by Reid Ewing for the Federal Highway Administration in 1999; he showed how the impact on traffic speed varies according to geometrics and spacing, whereas the impact on traffic volume is more related to the availability and quality of alternative routes.[47] Portland, Oregon, once suffering from heavy traffic congestion, was the first city to undertake a comprehensive master plan implementing 800 traffic-calming devices. These were added to 221 miles of bikeways that allowed pedestrians and cyclists to commute safely to downtown. Among the 100 largest cities in the United States, Portland was rated number one in meeting key Healthy People 2000 goals.[48]

ENFORCE TRAFFIC LAWS

A newly designed walkable community would not succeed without strict law enforcement to help drivers, bikers, and pedestrians coexist harmoniously with each other. Not much has been done until now to protect bikers and pedestrians from driving aggression. Enforcing speed limits in urban and residential areas could help reduce biking and pedestrian casualties and encourage the practice of these activities. Speed management seems to offer the greatest potential for injury prevention in residential areas with a lot of children.[49] In countries like Germany and the Netherlands, traffic regulations strongly favor pedestrians and bicyclists. Not stopping for pedestrians at crosswalks is considered a serious offense. Laws are also more strict for pedestrians and cyclists.[50]

Since bicycling is a mode of transportation, cyclists should be considered road users just like car drivers and should follow the same traffic rules. Traffic-safety education should be provided to children early in life to make them aware not only of the dangers of the street, but of their responsibilities as users. Pucher and Djikstra reported that in the Netherlands and Germany, all elementary schoolchildren receive extensive instructions on safe bicycling and walking practices, including traffic regulations, defensive walking and bicycling, and how to anticipate dangerous situations and react appropriately.[51] The current emphasis on helmet wearing as if it were the main solution to safety prevents the implementation of a real policy for biking as a mode of transportation.

24

The Route to Health

There is no doubt that the current level of physical inactivity is not going to decrease based only on individual solutions and willpower, or even with promotion programs targeting more vulnerable groups. Our immediate environment needs major changes to elicit a healthier lifestyle. Understanding the evolutionary importance of biped posture and locomotion for the human species and how the built environment has reduced the opportunity—and the ability—to walk in the second half of the twentieth century may help target the right avenues to solve the problem. Emphasizing the adverse consequences of not walking on health, social life, and financial impact should increase public awareness as well. But it would be a mistake to believe there is a single solution.

Coupled with healthier eating, exercising more during our daily routine is now a survival necessity. Because it keeps us physically active, walking can even act as a deterrent to constant food ingestion. Changing attitudes is the most effective way to promote walking: walking should become trendy, rather than being seen as dangerous or as a sign of low status. Walking has to be seen as a good way to preserve autonomy and independence, as a symbol of freedom, fitness, and a better quality of life. Increased mobility for the elderly, the poor, and the young should bring more freedom into their lives and decrease the burden on those who now act as their chauffeurs.

Efforts have to be made at different levels to reduce health threats:

- federal funding focusing on walkability of cities instead of new highways
- changes in zoning laws to allow mixed-use neighborhoods
- restrictions on low-density development and parking requirements
- subsidies to employees commuting to work by transit
- tax breaks for fitness programs
- increased physical education in schools
- walking prescriptions from health-care professionals
- more parks, sidewalks, bike lanes, and walking paths
- better public transit systems
- roads designed not only for cars but for pedestrians as well
- reallocation of existing road space to pedestrians

What is needed is a set of public policies that aim to enhance the walkability of communities and publicize the improvements that have been made. Walkable environments could also be promoted through the creation of walking clubs and the provision of walking-path maps. Incentives and opportunities have a better chance than education programs to inspire people to become more physically active.

Walking allows people to take control of the streets and makes them feel and be safer and healthier as individuals and collectively. Walking benefits them financially, because they do not have to pay for the adverse consequences of a sedentary lifestyle and a car-oriented way of life. Restoring a walkable environment is the best way to increase the fitness level of the population as a whole, because under such circumstances, everyone benefits from it. Compared to recreational walking, utilitarian walking is something you do not have to choose; the environment provides the opportunity. It is also a good way to achieve greater equity among individuals and social groups. Walking keeps people in closer touch with the environment, increasing their respect for it and their concern for its welfare. Walking also brings people closer to their fellow citizens.

Walking may not cure all health problems or city problems, but it can surely improve the current disastrous situation.

Epilogue

This book was written during my free time, which means that after sitting all day in front of my computer at work, I had to sit in front of my home computer at night working on the manuscript for about two years. There was not much time left for walking or even for cooking. It gave me the opportunity to personally experience what I was warning about. Beyond scientific facts, I can now tell you from personal experience that the sedentary lifestyle is harmful and will soon leave us handicapped if we do not react soon to this state of passiveness.

Selected Internet Resources on Walking and Walkable Communities

Here is a list of online resources providing useful tools to help individuals traveling on foot as part of their daily routine or helping their community restore a walkable environment.

WALKING AND CYCLING

America on the Move is a national imitative to help individuals and communities make positive changes to improve health and quality of life. The idea is to restore energy balance by eating less (100 fewer calories every day) and walking an extra 2,000 steps (about one mile) to prevent weight gain. Participants wear a pedometer to determine their daily count of steps. A goal of 10,000 daily steps is required to lose weight.
www.americaonthemove.org

America Walks is a national coalition of local advocacy groups dedicated to promoting walkable communities. Its mission is to foster the development of community-based pedestrian advocacy groups, educate the public about the benefits of walking, and act as a collective voice for walking advocates. The group is also involved in the preparation of the International Walk to School Day every year, and in the National Congress of Pedestrian Advocates.
www.americawalks.org

A useful resource for those who do not want to walk alone or whose neighborhood is not suitable for walking, the **American Volkssport Association** is a network of 350 walking clubs that organizes more than 3,000 walking events per year in all fifty states, as well as occasional biking, skiing, and swimming events. The walking event calendar for each state is available online.
www.ava.org

Go for Green—The Active Living and Environmental Program is a Canadian nonprofit organization whose mission is to encourage outdoor physical activity that protects, enhances, or restores the environment. Their program includes partnerships on a local, regional, and national basis to help Canadians improve their health and the health of the environment. Since 1992, they have supported more than 3,000 initiatives.
www.goforgreen.ca

The **League of American Bicyclists** represents the interests of the nation's fifty-seven million cyclists and works to bring better bicycling to the community by encouraging communities to provide better facilities for bicyclists, influencing transportation policy and legislation, and helping people feel more secure about getting on their bikes. It also identifies and designates bicycle-friendly communities.
www.bikeleague.org

The mission of the **National Center for Bicycling and Walking** is to create bicycle-friendly and walkable communities. The center provides specialized consulting services in planning, policy development, public involvement, and route selection; other activities include planning and design guidelines for bicycle and pedestrian facilities, training programs for public health and transportation agencies, economic development and tourism planning and analysis, and organizing and managing workshops and conferences.
www.bikewalk.org

The **National Coalition for Promoting Physical Activity** is a group of national organizations whose mission is to unite the strengths of public, private, and industry efforts in collaborative partnerships that inspire and empower Americans to lead more physically active lifestyles.
www.ncppa.org

The Pedestrian and Bicycle Information Center offers a huge amount of resources to make your community walkable. It provides a neighborhood walking guide and a walkability checklist to improve walkability. It gives a list of bicycle clubs and their Web links. It illustrates the health, transportation, environmental, and economic benefits of walking. Here you can obtain the *Pedestrian Facilities Users Guide*, published by the Federal Highway Administration in 2002, which can be useful for transportation engineers, planners, and safety professionals involved in increasing pedestrian safety and mobility. Citizens may also use it for identifying tools to improve the safety and mobility in their neighborhoods.
www.walkinginfo.org

Founded in 1986, the purpose of **Rails-to-Trails Conservancy** is to enrich America's communities and countryside by creating a nationwide network of public trails from former rail lines and connecting corridors. It has now reached 12,648 miles of rail-trails and around 100 million users per year. Rail-trails provide places for cyclists, hikers, walkers, runners, inline skaters, cross-country skiers, and physically challenged individuals to exercise and experience the wonders of the nation's urban, suburban, and rural environments, thus helping improve public health.
www.railtrails.org

Safe Routes to Schools is a movement that focuses on getting kids back on their feet and onto their bikes. It involves neighborhood groups, public health advocates, traffic engineers, and local officials in making streets safer along school routes. All the information on this program is provided by **Transportation Alternatives**, whose mission is to encourage bicycling, walking, and public transit as alternatives to automobile use. The organization is also a great source of information on traffic calming.
www.saferoutestoschools.org

Shape Up America is a national initiative to promote healthy weight and increased physical activity. Its purpose is to educate the public on the importance of the achievement and maintenance of a healthy body weight through the adoption of increased physical activity and healthy eating, based on the scientific evidence that obesity is not just an aesthetic problem but a condition that can lead to serious disease. Through health messages, it encourages small lifestyle changes that provide immediate health benefits.
www.shapeup.org

Walk and Bike to School promotes bicycling and walking to school through Walk to School events (first week of October) and Safe Routes to School programs, which enable children to incorporate physical activity into their daily routine to fight health problems related to inactivity, improve air quality, and make routes safer.
www.walktoschool.org

WALKABLE COMMUNITIES

The **Active Living Network** is part of a coordinated response to find creative approaches for integrating physical activity into American life. Rather than addressing obesity only, it focuses on how the built environment can promote more active lives.
www.activeliving.org

The **Center for Livable Communities (Local Government Commission)** is a nonprofit organization providing inspiration, technical assistance, and networking to local elected officials and other dedicated community leaders who are working to create healthy, walkable, and resource-efficient communities. The site provides information on community design, economic development, energy, environment, and transportation issues.
www.lgc.org

The **Congress for the New Urbanism** is a Chicago nonprofit organization involved in the creation of cities and towns based on mixed-use, walkable neighborhoods and attractive civic spaces. The site provides a good illustration of the group's principles.
www.cnu.org

The **Michigan Land Use Institute** was founded in 1995 to establish an approach to economic development that strengthens communities, enhances opportunity, and protects the state's unmatched natural resources. It is among the ten largest state-based Smart Growth and environmental advocacy organizations in the nation. The **Elm Street Writers Group** writes critiques of sprawl and city planning.
www.mlui.org

Partnership for a Walkable America is a national coalition working to improve the conditions for walking and to increase the number of Americans who walk regularly. The members are national governmental agencies and nonprofit organizations concerned with safety, health, and the environment. **www.walkableamerica.org**

Project for Public Spaces is a nonprofit organization in New York dedicated to creating and sustaining public places that build communities. It provides technical assistance, education, and research through programs in parks, plazas, and central squares; buildings and civic architecture; transportation; and public markets. The Web site provides books, videos, and an image collection of nearly one million photographs to help create great public spaces. **www.pps.org**

The **Sierra Club** is an environmental organization providing resources for citizens who want to promote smart growth. It emphasizes the adverse effects of sprawl and illustrates Smart Growth success stories in all fifty states. It also provides online computer-generated simulations showing the difference between sprawl and smart growth, demonstrating how sprawling communities can be revitalized and made more livable. **www.sierraclub.org**

Smart Growth America is a coalition of advocacy organizations that have a stake in how metropolitan expansion affects the environment, quality of life, and economic sustainability. It supports the type of growth that preserves farmland and open space, revitalizes neighborhoods, keeps housing affordable, ensures social equity, and provides more transportation choices. **www.smartgrowthamerica.com**

Smart Growth Online deals with issues related to smart growth such as community quality of life, design, economics, environment, health, housing, and transportation. The site provides a huge amount of documentation and resources in these areas. **www.smartgrowth.org**

The **Surface Transportation Policy Project** is a nationwide coalition working to ensure safer communities and smarter transportation choices that enhance the economy, improve public health, promote social equity, and protect the environment. It provides a series of reports dealing with these issues that help restore the livability of communities. **www.transact.org**

The **Victoria Transport Policy Institute**, located in Victoria, B.C., Canada, is dedicated to finding innovative solutions to transportation problems and land-use management. Its approach considers the economic, health, and environmental impacts of transportation policies. It also addresses the issues of safe walking and bicycling. A huge reference list on these subjects is available online.
www.vtpi.org

Walkable Communities is a nonprofit organization established in the state of Florida in 1996 that helps communities become more walkable and pedestrian friendly. It documents characteristics of such communities and provides a list of North American walkable places.
www.walkable.org

ILLUSTRATION CREDITS

Guy Langlois: photographs pages 5, 9, 53, 65, 74, 76, 79, 83, 91, 157, 159, 165, 167, 171, 174, 177, 178, 181.

Marie Demers: photograph page 67.

Copyright 2005 Project for Public Spaces, www.pps.org: two cover photographs; photographs pages 60, 186; figures pages 144, 150.

Todd Litman, If Health Matters, Victoria, BC: Victoria Transport Policy Institute, 2004 (data source: Centers for Disease Control and Prevention, National Center of Health Statistics, "Deaths: Preliminary Data for 2001," National Vital Statistics Reports 51:5, 14 March 2003, www.cdc.gov /nchs): graph, page 21.

John Pucher and John I. Renne, "Socioeconomics of Urban Travel: Evidence from the 2001 NHTS," Transportation Quarterly 57 (2003): 49–77: graphs on pages 30, 82.

John Pucher and L. Dijkstra, "Promoting Safe Walking and Cycling to Improve Public Health: Lessons from the Netherlands and Germany," American Journal of Public Health, 93 (2003): 1509-1516: graph on page 68.

World Health Organization, Health and Development Through Physical Activity and Sport, Geneva, 2003: figure on page 148.

NOTES

2 A WALKABLE HAVEN

1. McLuhan, *Understanding Media.*
2. Ewing et al., "Measuring Sprawl and Its Impact."
3. Holtz Kay, *Asphalt Nation.*
4. Ibid., 507.

3 A FEW STEPS BACK... IN HUMAN EVOLUTION

1. Reichholf, *L'émergence de l'homme.*
2. Clark, "Cycle Fit."
3. Holtz Kay, *Asphalt Nation.*
4. Killingsworth, "Health Promoting Community Design."
5. Frank et al., *Health and Community Design.*
6. Frumkin, "Urban Sprawl and Public Health."
7. Swinburn et al., "Obesogenic Environments."
8. Tyre, "Extra Pounds."
9. Koplan and Dietz, "Caloric Imbalance."
10. Ibid., 1580.
11. Roberts et al., "Pedalling Health."
12. Obesity Calendar: 2003: January 7, *San Francisco Chronicle*, www. defeatdiabetes.org/Articles/obesity030107.htm; February 2, CBSNews, www.cbsnews.com/stories/2003/02/06/health/main539710.shtml; March 27, Center for the Advancement of Health, www.hbns.org/ news/neighb03-27-03.cfm; April 30, Diabetes in Control.com, www.defeatdiabetes.org/Articles/television030430.htm; May 5, CBSNews, www.cbsnews.com/stories/2003/04/08/health/main548286.shtml; June 9, *Columbia* (MO) *Daily Tribune*, www.showmenews.com/2003/Jun/ 20030609Spor021.asp; July 30, ABCNews, www.discussionforums.us/ forum/archive/index.php/t-968.html; August 25, Helen Gibson, *Time*; September 7, ABCNews, www.hon.ch/News/HSN/511141.html; October 13, Associated Press; wcco.com/health/health_story_286145350.html; November 10, *NewScientist* News Service, www.newscientist.com/ news/news.jsp?id=ns99994364; December 22, *Oakland Tribune*, www.findarticles.com/p/articles/mi_qn4176/is_20031222/ai_n14560271. 2004: January 21, Associated Press, nature.berkeley.edu/pipermail/ prc-obesity-network-cwh/2004-January/000017.html; February 11, CTVNews, www.ctv.ca/servlet/ArticleNews/story/CTVNews/ 1076428936008_24; March 9, Associated Press, www.totalobscurity. com/mind/news/2004/eating-selves.htm; April 23, CBSNews, www.cbsnews.com/stories/2004/04/23/health/main613336.shtml; May

27, BBCNews, news.bbc.co.uk/1/hi/health/3752597.stm; June 15, *Fort Frances Times*, www.fftimes.com/index.php/3/2004-06-15/16857; July 1, *Medical News Today*, www.medicalnewstoday.com/medicalnews. php?newsid=10140; August 23, CBSNews, www.cbsnews.com/stories/ 2004/08/23/health/ main637912.shtml; September 21, *Medical News Today*, www.medicalnewstoday.com/medicalnews.php?newsid=13744; October 2, CTVNews, www.ctv.ca/servlet/ArticleNews/story/CTVNews/ 1096657306818_92066506?s_na...; November 5, *Medical News Today*, www.medicalnewstoday.com/medicalnews.php?newsid=15922; December 16, News-Medical.Net, www.news-medical.net/?id=6877.

13. Sturm, "Clinically Severe Obesity in the United States."
14. Schmidt, "Weighty Issue for Children."
15. Critser, *Fat Land.*
16. Mumford, *City in History.*

4 TRYING TO WALK IN THE UNITED STATES

1. Staples, "Most Dangerous Pedestrian in Los Angeles."

5 THE VALUE OF WALKING, AND THE PRICE OF NOT WALKING

1. Mumford, *City in History*, 507.
2. Cardinal, "Vélo, boulot, dodo."
3. Illich. *Energy and Equity.*
4. Kappelman, *Marshall McLuhan.*
5. Litman, "Economic Value of Walkability."
6. Solnit, *Wanderlust.*
7. Ibid., 260–261.
8. Ibid.

6 THE CONSPIRACY

1. "Obesity Industry."
2. Poston and Foreyt, "Obesity Is an Environmental Issue."

7 UNDERESTIMATING THE PROBLEM: THE VICTIMS

1. Pucher, "Transportation Paradise."
2. Brown, "Year of Living Statistically."
3. Lucy. "Mortality Risk Associated with Leaving Home."
4. Jedwab. "Getting to Work."
5. Ewing et al., "Urban Sprawl and Physical Activity."
6. McCann and Ewing, "Health Effects of Sprawl."
7. Ewing et al., "Measuring Sprawl and Its Impact."
8. Victoria Transport Policy Institute, *Transportation Demand Management Encyclopedia.*

9. Friedman et al., "Effect of Neotraditional Neighborhood Design."

10. Koplan and Dietz, "Caloric Imbalance and Public Health Policy."

11. Ernst and McCann, "Mean Streets 2002."

12. McCann and DeLille, "Mean Streets 2000."

13. The Pedestrian Danger Index is available for metro areas over one million residents in Ernst and McCann, "Mean Streets 2002."

14. Frumkin. "Urban Sprawl and Public Health."

15. Ernst and McCann, "Mean Streets 2002."

16. McCann and DeLille, "Mean Streets 2000."

17. Frank et al., *Health and Community Design.*

18. Roberts et al., "Urban Traffic Environment."

19. Roberts et al., "Driveway-Related Child Pedestrian Injuries."

20. Roberts et al., "Effect of Environmental Factors."

21. Stevenson et al., "Case-Control Study."

22. Roberts and Crombie, "Child Pedestrian Deaths."

23. Roberts et al., "Urban Traffic Environment."

24. Roberts et al., "Urban Traffic Environment."

25. Agran et al., "Role of the Physical and Traffic Environment."

26. Roberts et al., "Effect of Environmental Factors."

27. Stevenson et al., "Case Control Study."

28. Roberts, "Child Pedestrian Death Rates."

29. Roberts, "International Trends."

30. Mueller et al., "Environmental Factors."

31. Agran et al., "Role of the Physical and Traffic Environment."

32. Mueller et al., "Environmental Factors."

33. Joly et al., "Geographical and Socio-Ecological Variations."

34. Centers for Disease Control and Prevention, "Childhood Pedestrian Deaths."

35. Laflamme and Diderichsen, "Social Differences."

36. Dougherty et al., "Social Class."

37. Wazana et al., "Child Pedestrians."

38. Durkin et al., "Traffic Injuries."

40. DiMaggio and Durkin, "Child Pedestrian Injury."

41. Lightstone et al., "Motor Vehicle Collisions."

42. Agran et al., "Child Pedestrian Injury Events."

43. Winn et al., "Pedestrian Injuries to Children."

44. Roberts, "Driveway-Related Child Pedestrian Injuries."

45. Holland et al., "Driveway Motor Vehicle Injuries."

46. Nadler et al., "Driveway Injuries in Children."

47. Centers for Disease Control and Prevention, "Fatal Car Trunk Entrapment."

48. Roberts, "International Trends."

49. Roberts and Coggan, "Blaming Children."

50. Koepsell et al., "Crosswalk Markings."
51. Langlois et al., "Characteristics of Older Pedestrians."
52. Bailey et al., "Issues of Elderly Pedestrians."
53. Coffin and Morrall, "Walking Speeds of Elderly Pedestrians."
54. Balfour and Kaplan, "Neighborhood Environment."
55. Takano et al., "Urban Residential Environments."
56. King et al., "Convenience of Destinations."
57. Clark, "Effect of Walking on Lower Body Disability."
58. Surface Transportation Policy Project, "High Mileage Moms."
59. Economic Commission for Europe, *Statistics of Road Traffic Accidents.*
60. Hart and Spivak, *Elephant in the Bedroom.*
61. Wilkinson and Jacobsen, "Why Transportation Is a Health Issue."
62. Evans, "New Traffic Safety Vision."
63. Holtz Kay, *Asphalt Nation.*
64. Frumkin, "Urban Sprawl and Public Health."
65. Lucy, "Leaving Home."
66. Ewing, "Urban Sprawl as a Risk Factor."
67. Surface Transportation Policy Project, "Transportation and Economic Prosperity."
68. Surface Transportation Policy Project, "Transportation and Biodiversity."
69. Barash, *Sociobiology and Behavior.*
70. Macionis and Parillo, *Cities and Urban Life.*
71. Ferguson, "Road Rage."
72. Duany et al., *Suburban Nation.*
73. Phillips, *City Lights.*
74. Surface Transportation Policy Project, "Aggressive Driving."
75. Pollard, "Going to Work."
76. Surface Transportation Policy Project, "Transportation and Economic Prosperity."
77. Koslowsky et al., *Commuting Stress.*
78. Surface Transportation Policy Project, "Transportation and Economic Prosperity."
79. Texas Transportation Institute, "2003 Urban Mobility Study."
80. Illich, "Energy and Equity."
81. Surface Transportation Policy Project, "Transportation Data."
82. Pollard, "Going to Work."
83. Surface Transportation Policy Project, "Transportation Data."
84. Pucher, "Renaissance of Public Transport."
85. Jedwab, "Getting to Work."
86. Surface Transportation Policy Project, "Transportation Data."
87. Pollard, "Policy Prescriptions."
88. Pucher, "Renaissance of Public Transport."

8 THE DECLINE IN WALKING

1. Rafferty et al., "Physical Activity Patterns Among Walkers."
2. McCann and DeLille, "Mean Streets 2000."
3. Ernst and McCann, "Mean Streets 2002."
4. Ewing et al., "Measuring Sprawl and Its Impact."
5. Moore, "City, Suburban Designs."
6. Jedwab, "Getting to Work."
7. Owen et al., "Understanding Environmental Influences on Walking."
8. Duany et al., *Suburban Nation*, 34.
9. Centers for Disease Control and Prevention, "Neighborhood Safety."
10. Berrigan and Troiano, "Urban Form and Physical Activity."
11. U.S. Department of Transportation, "National Bicycling and Walking Study."
12. Brownson et al., "Determinants of Physical Activity."
13. Giles-Corti and Donovan, "Determinants of Physical Activity."
14. Giles-Corti and Donovan, "Socioeconomic Status Differences."
15. Giles-Corti and Donovan, "Correlates of Walking."
16. Ball, "Perceived Environmental Aesthetics."
17. Catlin et al., "Factors Associated with Overweight."
18. Giles-Corti et al., "Factors Associated with Overweight."
19. Craig et al., "Effect of the Environment on Physical Activity."
20. Victoria Transport Policy Institute, *Transportation Demand Management Encyclopedia.*
21. Ernst and McCann, "Mean Streets 2002."
22. McCann and DeLille, "Mean Streets 2000."
23. Transportation Research Board, "Risks of School Travel."
24. Duany et al., *Suburban Nation.*
25. Centers for Disease Control and Prevention, "Children Walking and Biking."
26. Centers for Disease Control and Prevention, "School Transportation Modes."
27. Roberts et al., "Exposure of Children to Traffic."
28. Litman, "Economic Value of Walkability."
29. Huttenmoser, "Children and Their Living Surroundings."
30. Ernst and McCann, "Mean Streets 2002."

9 THE CHALLENGE OF BICYCLING

1. Franklin, "Effectiveness of Cycle Helmets."
2. Robinson, "Bicycle Helmet Laws."
3. Franklin, "Effectiveness of Cycle Helmets."
4. Wardlaw, "Lessons for a Better Cycling Future."
5. Economic Commission for Europe, *Statistics of Road Traffic Accidents.*

6. Kifer, "Is Cycling Dangerous?"
7. Roberts et al., "Pedalling Health."
8. Ibid.
9. Clark, "Cycle Fit."
10. Wardlaw, "Lessons for a Better Cycling Future."
11. Holtz Kay, *Asphalt Nation.*
12. Pucher and Dijkstra, "Safe Walking and Cycling."
13. Clark, "Cycle Fit."
14. Pucher and Dijkstra, "Safe Walking and Cycling."
15. Clark, "Cycle Fit."
16. Holtz Kay, *Asphalt Nation.*
17. Pucher and Dijkstra, "Safe Walking and Cycling."
18. Pucher et al., "Bicycling Renaissance."
19. U.S. Department of Transportation, "National Bicycling and Walking Study," 46.
20. Pucher et al., "Bicycling Renaissance."
21. Frank et al., *Health and Community Design.*

10 DESTROYING THE LANDSCAPE

1. McLuhan, *Understanding Media,* 224.
2. Holtz Kay, *Asphalt Nation.*
3. Hart and Spivak, *Elephant in the Bedroom.*
4. Litman, "Transportation Land Use Impacts."
5. Surface Transportation Policy Project, "Transportation and Biodiversity."
6. Dannenberg et al., "Community Design and Land-Use Choices."
7. Sierra Club, "Sprawl."
8. Breunig, "Losing Ground."
9. Surface Transportation Policy Project California, "Traffic Congestion and Sprawl."
10. Sierra Club, "Sprawl."
11. Mid-Atlantic Integrated Assessment, "Urban Sprawl."
12. Sierra Club, "Sprawl."
13. Beck et al., "Outsmarting Smart Growth."
14. Macionis and Parillo, *Cities and Urban Life.*
15. Vellinga, "Dream Homes or Rural Nightmares?"
16. Kunstler, *Home from Nowhere.*
17. Kunstler, "Home from Nowhere."
18. Holtz Kay, *Asphalt Nation.*
19. Farrington, "Garage Door Dangers."
20. Kriel et al., "Hazard for Children."
21. Lofland, *Public Realm,* 232.
22. Litman, "Costs of Automobile Dependency."

23. Macaluso, "Link Between Health and Sprawl."
24. Surface Transportation Policy Project, "Why Are the Roads So Congested?"
25. Duany et al., *Suburban Nation*, 89.
26. Cited in Surface Transportation Policy Project California, "Traffic Congestion and Sprawl."
27. Mumford, *City in History*.
28. Ibid.
29. Kunstler, *Home from Nowhere*.

11 STREET DEMOCRACY IN JEOPARDY

1. Rudovsky, *Streets for People*.
2. Holtz Kay, *Asphalt Nation*.
3. Litman, "Costs of Automobile Dependency."
4. Ibid.
5. Surface Transportation Policy Project, "Transportation Costs."
6. McCann and Ewing, "Health Effects of Sprawl."
7. Frumkin, "Urban Sprawl and Public Health."
8. Duany et al., *Suburban Nation*.

12 THE VANISHING OF SOCIAL COHESION

1. Lofland, *Public Realm*.
2. Madanipour, *Design of Urban Space*.
3. Holtz Kay, *Asphalt Nation*.
4. Duany et al., *Suburban Nation*, 60.
5. Solnit, *Wanderlust*, 255.
6. Mumford, *City in History*, 512.
7. Putnam, *Bowling Alone*.
8. Leyden, "Social Capital and the Built Environment."
9. Putnam, *Bowling Alone*.
10. Kunstler, *Home from Nowhere*.
11. Blakely and Snyder, *Fortress America*.
12. Putnam, *Bowling Alone*.
13. Sampson et al., "Neighborhoods and Violent Crime."
14. Jacobs, *Death and Life of Great American Cities*, 56.
15. Paulos and Goodman, "Familiar Stranger Project."
16. Solnit, *Wanderlust*, 218.

13 TRAFFIC AIR POLLUTION

1. Kunzli et al., "Breathless in Los Angeles."
2. Surface Transportation Policy Project, "Transportation and the Environment."
3. Frumkin, "Urban Sprawl and Public Health."

4. Surface Transportation Policy Project, "Transportation and the Environment," "Transportation and Health."
5. Frumkin, "Urban Sprawl and Public Health."
6. Weinhold, "Don't Breathe and Drive?"
7. Ewing et al., "Measuring Sprawl and Its Impact."
8. Ernst et al., "Clearing the Air."
9. Beck et al., "Outsmarting Smart Growth."
10. Ernst et al., "Clearing the Air."
11. Frank et al., "Linking Land Use with Household Vehicle Emissions."
12. Jaffe et al., "Emergency Department Visits for Asthma."
13. Tolbert, et al., "Air Quality and Paediatric Emergency Room Visits."
14. Norris et al., "Fine Particles and Asthma Emergency Department Visits."
15. Committee of the Environmental and Occupational Health Assembly of the American Thoracic Society, "Health Effects of Outdoor Air Pollution."
16. Dockery et al., "Air Pollution and Mortality."
17. Burnett et al., "Urban Ambient Air Pollution Mix."
18. "Study Shows Massive Tree Loss."
19. Ibid.
20. Friedman et al., "Transportation and Commuting Behaviors."
21. Duhme et al., "Asthma and Allergic Rhinitis."
22. Weiland et al, "Wheezing and Allergic Rhinitis in Children."
23. Wjst et al., "Road Traffic."
24. Ciccone et al., "Road Traffic."
25. Van Vliet et al., "Chronic Respiratory Symptoms in Children."
26. Brunekreef et al., "Truck Traffic and Lung Function."
27. Edwards et al., "Hospital Admissions for Asthma."
28. Wilhelm and Ritz, "Adverse Birth Outcomes."

14 THE DECLINE IN PHYSICAL ACTIVITY

1. Sanmartin et al, "Canada/United States Survey of Health."
2. Roberts et al., "Pedalling Health."
3. Allied Dunbar National Fitness Survey, "Activity Patterns and Fitness Levels."
4. Adler, "Takeout Nation."
5. "Cut the Fat."
6. Centers for Disease Control and Prevention, "Prevalence of Physical Activity."
7. Ebbeling et al., "Childhood Obesity."
8. Ewing et al., "Urban Sprawl and Physical Activity."
9. Powell and Blair, "Sedentary Living Habits."
10. Colditz, "Costs of Obesity and Inactivity."

11. Vita et al., "Aging, Health Risks, and Cumulative Disability."
12. Katzmarzyk et al., "Physical Inactivity in Canada."
13. Greendale et al., "Leisure Exercise and Osteoporosis."
14. Prentice and Jebb, "Obesity in Britain."
15. Martinez-Gonzalez et al., "Physical Inactivity, Sedentary Lifestyle and Obesity."
16. Ball et al., "Too Fat to Exercise?"
17. Surface Transportation Policy Project, "Transportation and Health."
18. U.S. Department of Health and Human Services, "Physical Activity and Health."
19. Sealy, "Just Do It."
20. Brownell and Battle Horgen, *Food Fight.*
21. "Vending Machine Controversy."
22. "Cut the Fat."
23. Ludwig et al., "Sugar-Sweetened Drinks and Childhood Obesity."
24. Luepker, "How Physically Active Are American Children?"
25. Henry, "Too Fat to Get Fit."
26. Campbell et al., "School Sports Bid to Fight Obesity."
27. Townsend and Campbell, "Britain's Battle of the Bulge."
28. Patc et al., "Physical Activity and Other Health Behaviors."
29. Trudeau et al., "Primary School Physical Education."

15 THE INCREASE IN OBESITY

1. "Researcher Links Obesity, Food Portions."
2. Creager, "America's New Diet."
3. Eberwine, "Globesity."
4. Mokdad et al., "Epidemics of Obesity and Diabetes."
5. Mokdad et al., "Obesity Epidemic in the United States."
6. Center on an Aging Society, "Obesity Among Older Americans."
7. Sturm, "Clinically Severe Obesity in the United States."
8. Peeters et al., "Obesity in Adulthood."
9. Fontaine et al., "Years of Life Lost Due to Obesity."
10. Ogden et al., "Prevalence and Trends in Overweight."
11. Ebbeling et al., "Childhood Obesity."
12. "Bad Eating Habits Start Near Age 2."
13. Schwimmer et al., "Health-related Quality of Life."
14. "Fat Like Me."
15. Heini and Weinsier, "Divergent Trends in Obesity."
16. Mokdad et al., "Epidemics of Obesity and Diabetes."
17. "Cut the Fat."
18. Barnard, "Breaking the Food Seduction."
19. Mokdad et al., "Epidemics of Obesity and Diabetes."

20. Kahn et al., "Prescription Weight Loss Pills."
21. DeNoon, "How Fat Is Your City?"
22. Cameron et al., "Overweight and Obesity in Australia."
23. Tremblay and Willms, "Body Mass Index of Canadian Children."
24. Nash, "Obesity Goes Global."
25. Visscher and Seidell, "Public Health Impact of Obesity."
26. Chopra et al., "Epidemic of Overnutrition."
27. French et al., "Eating and Physical Activity."
28. Revill, "Deadly Slice of American Pie."
29. Jebb and Moore, "Sedentary Lifestyle and Inactivity."
30. Creager, "America's New Diet."
31. "Cut the Fat."
32. Robinson, *Consumer Reports.*

16 OBESITY AND HEALTH
 1. Must et al., "Overweight and Obesity."
 2. Visscher and Seidell, "Public Health Impact of Obesity."
 3. Gustafson et al., "Overweight and Risk of Alzheimer Disease."
 4. Field et al., "Impact of Overweight."
 5. Ibid.
 6. Koplan and Dietz, "Caloric Imbalance and Public Health Policy."
 7. Elias et al., "Lower Cognitive Function."
 8. Sturm, "Obesity, Smoking, and Drinking."
 9. Hussain, "Hospitals Buy More Extra-Large Gear."
10. Finkelstein, "National Medical Spending."
11. Daviglus et al., "Body Mass Index in Middle Age."
12. "US Kids Show Early Signs of Heart Disease."
13. Gorman, "Why So Many Are Getting Diabetes."
14. Visscher and Seidell, "Public Health Impact of Obesity."
15. Lakdawalla et al., "Are the Young Becoming More Disabled?"
16. Visscher and Seidell, "Public Health Impact of Obesity."
17. Calle et al., "Overweight, Obesity, and Mortality from Cancer."
18. Mokdad et al., "Epidemics of Obesity and Diabetes."
19. Centers for Disease Control and Prevention, "Prevalence of Diabetes."
20. Eberwine, "Globesity."
21. Cameron et al., "Overweight and Obesity in Australia."
22. Wolf and Colditz, "Cost of Obesity in the United States."
23. Visscher and Seidell, "Public Health Impact of Obesity."
24. Narayan et al., "Lifetime Risk for Diabetes Mellitus."
25. Diamond, "Double Puzzle."
26. Gorman, "Why So Many Are Getting Diabetes."
27. Mokdad et al., "Actual Causes of Death in the United States."

28. Calle et al., "Body-mass Index and Mortality."
29. "Obesity Factfile."
30. Allison et al., "Annual Deaths Attributable to Obesity."
31. Thompson, "Pets Mirror Nation's Obesity Problem."
32. Diamond, "Double Puzzle."

17 THE COSTS OF OBESITY

1. Colditz, "Costs of Obesity and Inactivity."
2. Wolf and Colditz, "Cost of Obesity in the United States."
3. Wang et al., "Cardiovascular Disease Associated with Excess Body Weight."
4. National Diabetes Information Clearinghouse, "National Diabetes Statistics."
5. Diamond, "Double Puzzle."
6. News-Medical.Net, "Diabetes set to Increase."
7. Seidell, "Costs of Obesity."
8. Lewis, "Overweight Workers."
9. Birmingham et al., "Cost of Obesity in Canada."
10. Thompson et al., "Costs of Obesity to U.S. Business."
11. Nolte et al., "U.S. Military Weight Standards."
12. Harrison et al., "Physical Activity Patterns."
13. Paris et al., "Type 2 Diabetes in the Military."
14. Robbins et al., "Body Weight Among Active Duty Personnel."

18 THE ROLE OF TELEVISION

1. French et al., "Eating and Physical Activity."
2. Dietz, "Role of Lifestyle in Health."
3. Putnam, Bowling Alone.
4. Kappelman, Marshall McLuhan.
5. Putnam, Bowling Alone.
6. Ibid.
7. Ibid., 237.
8. Prentice and Jebb, "Obesity in Britain."
9. Gallo, "Food Advertising in the United States."
10. French et al., "Eating and Physical Activity."
11. Babula, "A Family Affair."
12. Tucker and Friedman, "Television Viewing and Obesity in Adult Males."
13. Tucker and Bagwell, "Television Viewing and Obesity in Adult Females."
14. Salmon et al., "Television Viewing and Overweight."
15. Cameron et al., "Overweight and Obesity in Australia."
16. Hu et al., "Physical Activity and Television Watching."
17. Hu et al., "Television Watching and Other Sedentary Behaviors."
18. Singer, "Role of Television."

19. Dietz and Gortmaker, "Obesity and Television Viewing."
20. Gortmaker et al., "Television Viewing As a Cause of Increasing Obesity."
21. Andersen et al., "Physical Activity and Television Watching."
22. Lowry et al., "Television Viewing and Its Associations."
23. Janz et al., "Fatness, Physical Activity, and Television Viewing."
24. Klesges et al., "Effects of Television on Metabolic Rate."
25. Robinson, "Television Viewing and Childhood Obesity."
26. Dietz, "Role of Lifestyle in Health."
27. Schmidt, "Weighty Issue for Children."
28. Putnam, *Bowling Alone.*
29. Dennison et al., "Television Viewing and Television in Bedroom."
30. Certain and Kahn, "Television Viewing Among Infants and Toddlers."
31. Bernard et al., "Toppled Television Sets."
32. DiScala et al., "Television Sets Toppling onto Toddlers."

20 ON YOUR FEET

1. Surface Transportation Policy Project, "Americans' Attitudes Toward Walking."
2. U.S. Department of Transportation, "National Bicycling and Walking Study."
3. Ibid.
4. Pedestrian and Bicycle Information Center, "Safe Walking and Bicycling."
5. Ibid.
6. Environics International, "1998 Survey on Active Transportation."
7. Williams-Derry, "Who Is the Smart Growth Leader?"

21 THE BENEFITS OF WALKING

1. Leden, "Pedestrian Risk Decrease with Pedestrian Flow."
2. Alvord, *Divorce Your Car!*
3. Ibid.
4. Pate et al., "Physical Activity and Public Health."
5. Morris and Hardman, "Walking to Health."
6. Kelley et al., "Walking and Resting Blood Pressure."
7. Moreau et al., "Increasing Daily Walking."
8. Wong et al., "Cardiorespiratory Fitness."
9. Slentz et al., "Effects of the Amount of Exercise."
10. Ibid.
11. Jakicic et al., "Effect of Exercise Duration and Intensity."
12. Manson et al., "Walking Compared with Vigorous Exercise."
13. Fox, "Influence of Physical Activity."
14. Paluska and Schwenk, "Physical Activity and Mental Health."
15. U.S. Department of Health and Human Services, "Physical Activity and Health."

16. Bassett et al., "Physical Activity in an Old Order Amish Community."
17. Feskanich et al., "Walking and Leisure-Time Activity."
18. Brach et al., "Community-Dwelling Older Women."
19. Morris and Hardman, "Walking to Health."
20. Gregg et al., "Relationship of Walking to Mortality."
21. Central Practice of Acupuncture and Chinese Medicine, "Constipations."
22. Derby et al., "Erectile Dysfunction."
23. U.S. Department of Health and Human Services, "Physical Activity and Health."
24. McTiernan et al., "Risk of Breast Cancer."
25. BBC News World Edition, "Breast Cancer Less Likely in Cyclists."
26. Fox, "Housework, Walking Lowers Cancer."
27. Clark, "Cycle Fit."
28. Laurin et al., "Cognitive Impairment and Dementia."
29. Abbott et al., "Walking and Dementia."
30. Weuve et al., "Cognitive Function in Older Women."
31. Lee and Paffenbarger, "Light, Moderate, and Vigorous Intensity Physical Activity."
32. Andersen et al., "Mortality Associated with Physical Activity."
33. Sparling et al., "Promoting Physical Activity."

22 INDIVIDUAL SOLUTIONS

1. Pate et al., "Physical Activity and Public Health."
2. Kennedy and Meeuwisse, "Exercise Counselling."
3. Manson et al., "Pandemics of Obesity and Sedentary Lifestyle."
4. Brownell and Battle Horgen, *Food Fight.*
5. Boutelle et al., "Stair Use in a Public Building."
6. Tanner, "Eating Ourselves to Death."
7. Bauman et al., "Epidemiology of Dog Walking."
8. O'Connor, "You and Your Canine Companion."
9. Rooney et al., "Is Knowing Enough?"
10. Iwane et al., "Walking 10,000 Steps/Day."
11. Bassett et al., "Measurement of Daily Walking Distance."
12. Nestle and Jacobson, "Halting the Obesity Epidemic."
13. Roberts et al., "Pedalling Health."
14. U.S. Department of Health and Human Services, "Physical Activity and Health."
15. Centers for Disease Control and Prevention, "Neighborhood Safety."

23 CREATING WALKABLE ENVIRONMENTS

1. Pollard, "Policy Prescriptions."
2. Macionis and Parillo, *Cities and Urban Life.*

3. Hirschhorn, "Zoning Should Promote Public Health."
4. Kersh and Morone, "Politics Of Obesity."
5. Creager, "America's New Diet."
6. Macionis and Perillo, *Cities and Urban Life.*
7. Victoria Transport Policy Institute, *Transportation Demand Management Encyclopedia.*
8. Ibid.
9. Gillham, *Limitless City.*
10. Cited in Pollard, "Policy Prescriptions."
11. Sierra Club, "Smart Choices."
12. Ibid.
13. Duany et al., *Suburban Nation.*
14. Bicycle Federation of America Campaign to Make America Walkable, "Creating Walkable Communities."
15. Duany et al., *Suburban Nation.*
16. Ibid.
17. Kunstler, "Home from Nowhere."
18. Moore, "City, Suburban Designs."
19. Zegeer et al., "Pedestrian Facilities Users Guide."
20. Pucher et al., "Bicycling Renaissance?"
21. French et al., "Eating and Physical Activity."
22. Pucher et al., "Bicycling Renaissance."
23. Harnik, "History of the Rail-Trail Movement."
24. French et al, "Eating and Physical Activity."
25. Merom et al., "Environmental Intervention to Promote Walking and Cycling."
26. American Discovery Trail Society, "News and Information."
27. Geller, "Smart Growth."
28. Sierra Club, "Sprawl."
29. Surface Transportation Policy Project, "Safe Routes to School Programs."
30. Pedestrian and Bicycle Information Center, "Growing Demand."
31. Surface Transportation Policy Project California, "Traffic Congestion and Sprawl."
32. Staunton et al., "Safe Walking and Biking to School."
33. Camph, "Transportation, the ISTEA, and American Cities."
34. Surface Transportation Policy Project, "Changing Direction."
35. Ibid.
36. Geller, "Smart Growth."
37. Sierra Club, "Smart Choices."
38. Holtz Kay, *Asphalt Nation.*
39. Wheatley, "London's Traffic Woes."
40. Mindell et al., "Health Impact Assessment."

41. Cited in Pollard, "Policy Prescriptions."
42. Cited in Retting et al., "Traffic Engineering Measures."
43. Retting et al., "Crash and Injury Reduction."
44. Local Government Commission Center for Livable Communities, "Economic Benefits of Walkable Communities."
45. Litman, "Traffic Calming Benefits."
46. Ibid.
47. Ewing, "Traffic Calming."
48. Geller, "Smart Growth."
49. Retting et al., "Traffic Engineering Measures."
50. Pucher and Dijkstra, "Safe Walking and Cycling."
51. Ibid.

BIBLIOGRAPHY

Abbott, R. D., L. R. White, G. W. Ross, et al. "Walking and Dementia in Physically Capable Elderly Men." *Journal of the American Medical Association* 292 (2004): 1447–1453.

Adler J. "Takeout Nation." *Newsweek*, 9 February 2004. www.msnbc.msn.com/id/4121245

Agran, P. F., D. G. Winn, and C. L. Anderson. "Differences in Child Pedestrian Injury Events by Location." *Pediatrics* 93 (1994): 284–288.

———."The Role of the Physical and Traffic Environment in Child Pedestrian Injuries." *Pediatrics* 98 (1996): 1096–1103.

Allied Dunbar National Fitness Survey. *A Report on Activity Patterns and Fitness Levels.* London: Sports Council and Health Education Authority, 1992.

Allison, D. B., K. R. Fontaine, J. E. Manson, et al. "Annual Deaths Attributable to Obesity in the United States." *Journal of the American Medical Association* 282 (1999): 1530–1538.

Alvord, K. *Divorce Your Car! Ending the Love Affair with the Automobile.* Gabriola Island, BC, Canada: New Society Publishers, 2000.

American Discovery Trail Society. "News and Information." 2005. www.discoverytrail.org/news/faqs.html

Andersen, L. B., P. Schnohr, M. Schroll, et al. "All-cause Mortality Associated with Physical Activity During Leisure Time, Work, Sports, and Cycling to Work." *Archives of Internal Medicine* 160 (2000): 1621–1628.

Andersen, R. E., C. J. Crespo, S. J. Bartlett, et al. "Relationship of Physical Activity and Television Watching with Body Weight and Level of Fatness Among Children." *Journal of the American Medical Association* 279 (1998): 938–942.

Babula, J. "A Family Affair: Years of Bad Habits Weigh Heavily on Health." *Las Vegas Review–Journal,* 22 June 2003. www.reviewjournal.com/lvrj_home/2003/Jun-22-Sun-2003/news/21582230.html

"Bad Eating Habits Start Near Age 2: Study." Associated Press, 27 October 2003. www.ctv.ca/servlet/ArticleNews/story/CTVNews/1067261195146_28

Bailey, S. S., S. A. Jones, R. J. Stout, et al. "Issues of Elderly Pedestrians." *Transportation Research Record* 1375 (1992): 68–73.

Balfour, J. L., and G. A. Kaplan. "Neighborhood Environment and Loss of Physical Function in Older Adults: Evidence from the Alameda County Study." *American Journal of Epidemiology* 155 (2002): 507–519.

Ball, K., A. Bauman, E. Leslie, et al. "Perceived Environmental Aesthetics and Convenience and Company Are Associated with Walking for Exercise Among Australian Adults." *Preventive Medicine* 33 (2001): 434–440.

Ball, K., D. Crawford, and N. Owen. "Too Fat to Exercise? Obesity As a Barrier to Physical Activity." *Australia and New Zealand Journal of Public Health* 24 (2000): 331–333.

Barash, D. P. *Sociobiology and Behavior.* New York: Elsevier, 1977.

Barnard, N. *Breaking the Food Seduction: The Hidden Reasons Behind Food Cravings and 7 Steps to End Them Naturally.* New York: St. Martin's Press, 2003.

Bassett, D. R. Jr., A. L. Cureton, and B. E. Ainsworth. "Measurement of Daily Walking Distance: Questionnaire Versus Pedometer." *Medicine and Science in Sports and Exercise* 32 (2000): 1018–1023.

Bassett, D. R. Jr., P. L. Schneider, and G. E. Huntington. "Physical Activity in an Old Order Amish Community." *Medicine and Science in Sports and Exercise* 36 (2004): 79–85.

Bauman, A. E., S. J. Russell, S. E. Furber, et al. "The Epidemiology of Dog Walking: An Unmet Need for Human and Canine Health." *Medical Journal of Australia* 175 (2001): 632–634.

Beck, R., L. Kolankiewicz, and S. A. Camarota. "Outsmarting Smart Growth: Population Growth, Immigration, and the Problem of Sprawl." Washington, DC: Center for Immigration Studies, 2003. www.cis.org/articles/2003/sprawl.html

Benfield, F. K., M. D. Raimi, and D. D. T. Chen. "Once There Were Greenfields: How Urban Sprawl Is Undermining America's Environment, Economy and Social Fabric." Washington, DC: Surface Transportation Policy Project, 1999.

Bernard, P. A., C. Johnston, S. E. Curtis, et al. "Toppled Television Sets Cause Significant Pediatric Morbidity and Mortality." *Pediatrics* 102 (1998): E32.

Berrigan, D., and R. P. Troiano. "The Association Between Urban Form and Physical Activity in U.S. Adults." *American Journal of Preventive Medicine* 23 (2002): 74–79.

Bicycle Federation of America Campaign to Make America Walkable. "Creating Walkable Communities: A Guide for Local Governments." Prepared for Mid-America Regional Council, Kansas City, MO, 1998. www.marc.org/cwctoc.pdf

Birmingham, C. L., J. L. Muller, A. Palepu, et al. "The Cost of Obesity in Canada." *Canadian Medical Association Journal* 160 (1999): 483–488.

Blakely, E. J., and M. G. Snyder. *Fortress America: Gated Communities in the United States.* Washington, DC: Brookings Institute Press, 1997.

Boutelle, K. N., R. W. Jeffery, D. M. Murray, et al. "Using Signs, Artwork, and Music to Promote Stair Use in a Public Building." *American Journal of Public Health* 91 (2001): 2004–2006.

Brach, J. S., S. FitzGerald, A. B. Newman, et al. "Physical Activity and Functional Status in Community-Dwelling Older Women." *Archives of Internal Medicine* 163 (2003): 2565–2571.

"Breast Cancer Less Likely in Cyclists." BBC News World Edition, 10 February 2003. news.bbc.co.uk/2/hi/health/2743965.stm

Breunig, K. "Losing Ground: At What Cost? Changes in Land Use and Their Impact on Habitat, Biodiversity, and Ecosystem Services in Massachusetts." Massachusetts Audubon Society, 2003. www.massaudubon.org/losingground

Brown, I. "The Year of Living Statistically." *Globe and Mail*, 31 May 2003.

Brownell, K. D., and K. Battle Horgen. *Food Fight: The Inside Story of the Food Industry, America's Obesity Crisis, and What We Can Do About It.* Chicago: Contemporary Books, 2004.

Brownson, R. C., E. A. Baker, R. A. Housemann, et al. "Environmental and Policy Determinants of Physical Activity in the United States." *American Journal of Public Health* 91 (2001): 1995–2003.

Brunekreef, B., N. A. H. Janssen, J. de Hartog, et al. "Air Pollution from Truck Traffic and Lung Function in Children Living Near Motorways." *Epidemiology* 8 (1997): 298–303.

Burnett, R. T., S. Cakmak, and J. R. Brook. "The Effect of the Urban Ambient Air Pollution Mix on Daily Mortality Rates in 11 Canadian Cities." *Canadian Journal of Public Health* 89 (1998): 152–156.

Calle, E. E., C. Rodriguez, K. Walker-Thurmond, et al. "Overweight, Obesity, and Mortality from Cancer in a Prospectively Studied Cohort of U.S. Adults." *New England Journal of Medicine* 348 (2003): 1625–1638.

Calle, E. E., M. J. Thun, J. M. Petrelli, et al. "Body-mass Index and Mortality in a Prospective Cohort of U.S. Adults." *New England Journal of Medicine* 341 (1999): 1097–1105.

Cameron, A.J., T. A. Wellborn, P. Z. Zimmet, et al. "Overweight and Obesity in Australia: The 1999–2000 Australian Diabetes, Obesity and Lifestyle Study (AusDiab)." *Medical Journal of Australia* 178 (2003): 427–432.

Campbell, D. C., M. Townsend, and J. Revill. "Stars Back School Sports Bid to Fight Obesity." *Observer*, 21 September 2003. observer.guardian.co.uk/uk_news/story/0,6903,1046641,00.html

Camph, D. H. "Transportation, the ISTEA, and American Cities." Washington, DC: Surface Transportation Policy Project Monograph Series, 1996. www.transact.org/report.asp?id=22

Cardinal, F. "Vélo, boulot, dodo." *La Presse, Montreal,* 5 June 2004.

Catlin, T. K., E. J. Simoes, and R. C. Brownson. "Environmental and Policy Factors Associated with Overweight Among Adults in Missouri." *American Journal of Health Promotion* 17 (2003): 249–258.

Center on an Aging Society. "Obesity Among Older Americans: Challenges for the 21st Century." Washington, DC: Georgetown University, no. 10, July 2003. ihcrp.georgetown.edu/agingsociety/pubhtml/obesity2/obesity2.html

Centers for Disease Control and Prevention. "Barriers to Children Walking and Biking to School: United States, 1999." *Morbidity and Mortality Weekly Report* 51 (2002): 701–704.

———. "Childhood Pedestrian Deaths During Halloween: United States, 1975–1996." *Morbidity and Mortality Weekly Report* 46 (1997): 987–990.

———. "Fatal Car Trunk Entrapment Involving Children: United States, 1987–1998." *Morbidity and Mortality Weekly Report* 47 (1998): 1019–1022.

———. "Neighborhood Safety and the Prevalence of Physical Inactivity: Selected States, 1996." *Morbidity and Mortality Weekly Report* 48 (1999): 143–147.

———. "Prevalence of Diabetes and Impaired Fasting Glucose in Adults: United States, 1999–2000." *Morbidity and Mortality Weekly Report* 52 (2003): 833–837.

———. "Prevalence of Physical Activity, Including Lifestyle Activities, Among Adults: United States, 2000–2001." *Morbidity and Mortality Weekly Report* 52 (2003): 764–769.

———. "School Transportation Modes: Georgia, 2000." *Morbidity and Mortality Weekly Report* 51 (2002): 704–705.

Central Practice Clinic of Acupuncture and Chinese Medicine, "Constipations." www.centralpractice.4mg.com/constipations.htm

Certain, L. K., and R. S. Kahn. "Prevalence, Correlates, and Trajectory of Television Viewing Among Infants and Toddlers." *Pediatrics* 109 (2002): 634–642.

Chopra, M., S. Galbraith, and I. Darnton-Hill. "A Global Response to a Global Problem: The Epidemic of Overnutrition." *Bulletin of the World Health Organization* 80 (2002): 952–958.

Ciccone, G., F. Forastiere, N. Agabiti, et al. "Road Traffic and Adverse Respiratory Effects in Children. SIDRIA Collaborative Group." *Occupational and Environmental Medicine* 58 (1998): 771–778.

Clapp, J. A. *The City: A Dictionary of Quotable Thought on Cities and Urban Life.* Piscataway, NJ: Transaction Publishers, 1984.

Clark, D. O. "The Effect of Walking on Lower Body Disability Among Older Blacks and Whites." *American Journal of Public Health* 86 (1996): 57–61.

Clark, J. S. "Cycle Fit." Brickbat, 2003. www.brickbats.co.uk/Articles/Health.html

Coffin, A., and J. Morrall. "Walking Speeds of Elderly Pedestrians at Crosswalks." *Transportation Research Record* 1487 (1996): 63–67.

Colditz, G. A. "Economic Costs of Obesity and Inactivity." *Medicine and Science in Sports and Exercise* 31 (1999): S663–S667.

Committee of the Environmental and Occupational Health Assembly of the American Thoracic Society. "Health Effects of Outdoor Air Pollution." *American Journal of Respiratory and Critical Care Medicine* 153 (1996): 3–50.

Craig, C. L., R. C. Brownson, S. E. Cragg, et al. "Exploring the Effect of the Environment on Physical Activity: A Study Examining Walking to Work." *American Journal of Preventive Medicine* 23 (2002): 36–43.

Creager, E. "Plan for America's New Diet: Less Sprawl, Less Fat, Less Frenzy." *Miami Herald,* 2 June 2003. www.activelivingleadership.org/news6.htm

———. "Seven Plans to Get America Moving." *Miami Herald,* 2 June 2003. www.shapenews.com

———. "Western-style Consumption Worldwide Fuels 'Globesity.'" *Miami Herald,* 2 June 2003. ww.shapenews.com

Critser, G. *Fat Land: How Americans Became the Fattest People in the World.* New York: Houghton Mifflin, 2003.

"Cut the Fat." *Consumer Reports,* January 2004, 12–16.

Dannenberg, A. L., R. J. Jackson, H. Frumkin, et al. "The Impact of Community Design and Land-Use Choices on Public Health: A Scientific Research Agenda." *American Journal of Public Health* 93 (2003): 1500–1508.

Daviglus, M. L., K. Liu, L. L. Yan, et al. "Body Mass Index in Middle Age and Health-related Quality of Life in Older Age." *Archives of Internal Medicine* 163 (2003): 2448–2455.

Dennison, B. A., T. A. Erb, and P. L. Jenkins. "Television Viewing and Television in Bedroom Associated with Overweight Risk Among Low-Income Pre-School Children." *Pediatrics* 109 (2002): 1028–1035.

DeNoon, D. "How Fat Is Your City?" WebMD Medical News, 7 January 2004. my.webmd.com/content/article/79/96113.htm

Derby, C. A., B. A. Mohr, I. Goldstein, et al. "Modifiable Risk Factors and Erectile Dysfunction: Can Lifestyle Changes Modify Risk?" *Urology* 56 (2000): 302–306.

"Diabetes Set to Increase from 177m Worldwide to 370m by 2030." News-Medical.Net, 4 April 2005. www.news-medical.net/?id=8924

Diamond, J. "The Double Puzzle of Obesity." *Nature* 423 (2003): 599–602.

Dietz, W. H. "The Role of Lifestyle in Health: The Epidemiology and Consequences of Inactivity." *Proceedings of the Nutrition Society* 55 (1996): 829–840.

———, and S. L. Gortmaker. "Do We Fatten Our Children at the Television Set? Obesity and Television Viewing in Children and Adolescents." *Pediatrics* 75 (1985): 807–812.

DiMaggio, C., and M. Durkin. "Child Pedestrian Injury in an Urban Setting: Descriptive Epidemiology." *Academy of Emergency Medicine* 9 (2002): 54–62.

DiScala, C., M. Barthel, and R. Sege. "Outcomes from Television Sets Toppling onto Toddlers." *Archives of Pediatric and Adolescence Medicine* 155 (2001): 145–148.

Dockery, D. W., C.A. Pope III, X. Xu, et al. "An Association Between Air Pollution and Mortality in Six U.S. Cities." *New England Journal of Medicine* 329 (1993): 1753–1759.

Dougherty, G., I. B. Pless, and R. Wilkins. "Social Class and the Occurrence of Traffic Injuries and Deaths in Urban Children." *Canadian Journal of Public Health* 81 (1990): 204–209.

Duany, A., E. Plater-Zyberk, and J. Speck. *Suburban Nation: The Rise of Sprawl and the Decline of the American Dream.* New York: North Point Press, 2000.

Duhme, H., S. K. Weiland, U. Keil, et al. "The Association Between Self-Reported Symptoms of Asthma and Allergic Rhinitis and Self-Reported Traffic Density on Street of Residence in Adolescents." *Epidemiology* 7 (1996): 578–582.

Durkin, M. S., D. Laraque, I. Lubman, et al. "Epidemiology and Prevention of Traffic Injuries to Urban Children and Adolescents." *Pediatrics* 103 (1999): e74.

Ebbeling, C. B., D. B. Pawlak, D. S. Ludwig. "Childhood Obesity: Public-Health Crisis, Common Sense Cure." *Lancet* 360 (2002): 473–482.

Eberwine, D. "Globesity: The Crisis of Growing Proportions." *Perspective in Health Magazine* 7 (2002): 1–8. www.paho.org/English/DPI/Number15_article2_5.htm

Economic Commission for Europe. *Statistics of Road Traffic Accidents in Europe and North America,* vol. 43. New York and Geneva: United Nations, 1998.

Edwards, J., S. Walters, and R. K. Griffiths. "Hospital Admissions for Asthma in Preschool Children: Relationship to Major Roads in Birmingham, United Kingdom." *Archives of Environmental Health* 49 (1994): 223–227.

Elias, M. F., P. K. Elias, L. M. Sullivan, et al. "Lower Cognitive Function in the Presence of Obesity and Hypertension: The Framingham Heart Study." *International Journal of Obesity* 27 (2003): 260–268.

Environics International. "National Survey on Active Transportation." Ottawa, ON, Canada: Go for Green, 1998. www.goforgreen.ca

Ernst, M., J. Corless, and R. Greene-Roesel. "Clearing the Air." Washington, DC: Surface Transportation Policy Project, 2003. www.transact.org/report.asp?id=228

Ernst, M., and B. McCann. "Mean Streets 2002." Washington, DC: Surface Transportation Policy Project, 2002. www.transact.org/report.asp?id=202

Evans, L. "A New Traffic Safety Vision for the United States." *American Journal of Public Health* 93 (2003): 1384–1386.

Ewing, R. "Traffic Calming: State of the Practice." Washington, DC: U.S. Department of Transportation, Federal Highway Administration, 1999, Report no. FHWA-RD-99-135. www.ite.org/traffic/tcstate.htm

Ewing, R., R. Pendall, and D. Chen. "Measuring Sprawl and Its Impact." Washington, DC: Smarth Growth America, 2002. www.smartgrowthamerica.org/sprawlindex.html

Ewing, R., R. A. Schieber, and C. V. Zegeer. "Urban Sprawl As a Risk Factor in Motor Vehicle Occupant and Pedestrian Fatalities." *American Journal of Public Health* 93 (2003): 1541–1545.

Ewing, R., T. Schmid, R. Killingsworth, et al. "Relationship Between Urban Sprawl and Physical Activity, Obesity, and Morbidity." *American Journal of Health Promotion* 18 (2003): 47–57.

Farrington, B. "Garage Door Dangers." Homestore.com, 2003. www.homestore.com/HomeGarden/GarageDriveway/GarageDoorDangers.asp

"Fat Like Me: How to Win the Weight War." ABCNews.com, 27 October 2003. DVD available for purchase at: www.abcnewsstore.com/store/index.cfm?fuseaction=customer. product&product_code=S031027%2001&category_code=5

Ferguson, A. "Road Rage: Aggressive Driving Is America's Car Sickness du Jour." *Time*, 12 January 1998.

Feskanich, D., W. Willett, and G. Colditz. "Walking and Leisure-time Activity and Risk of Hip Fracture in Postmenopausal Women." *Journal of the American Medical Association* 288 (2002): 2300–2306.

Field, A. E., E. H. Coakley, A. Must, et al. "Impact of Overweight on the Risk of Developing Common Chronic Diseases During a 10-Year Period." *Archives of Internal Medicine* 161 (2001): 1581–1586.

Finkelstein, E. A., I. C. Fiebelkorn, and G. Wang. "National Medical Spending Attributable to Overweight and Obesity: How Much, and Who's Paying?" *Health Affairs* (January–June 2003): suppl Web exclusives: W3-219–226.

Fontaine, K. R., D. T. Redden, C. Wang, et al. "Years of Life Lost Due to Obesity." *Journal of the American Medical Association* 289 (no. 2, 2003): 187–193.

Fox, K. R. "The Influence of Physical Activity on Mental Well-Being." *Public Health Nutrition* 2 (1999): 411–418.

Fox, M. "Study: Housework, Walking Lowers Cancer, Death Risk." Yahoo! News, 2004. www.naturalsolutionsradio.com/articles/article.html?id=9492&filter=

Frank, L. D., and P. O. Engelke. "How Land Use and Transportation Systems Impact Public Health: A Literature Review of the Relationship Between Physical Activity and Built Form." Active Community Environments Initiative Working Paper, no. 1, 2001.

Frank, L. D., P. O. Engelke, and T. L. Schmid. *Health and Community Design: The Impact of the Built Environment on Physical Activity.* Washington, DC: Island Press, 2003.

Frank, L. D., B. Stone, and W. Bachman. "Linking Land Use with Household Vehicle Emissions in the Central Puget Sound: Methodological Framework and Findings," in *Transportation Research*, Part D. New York: Elsevier Science, 2000, 173–196.

Franklin, J. "The Effectiveness of Cycle Helmets." Calgary, AL, Canada: Elbow Valley Cycle Club, 2003. www.elbowvalleycc.org/helmetrp.html

French, S. A., M. Story, and R. W. Jeffery. "Environmental Influences on Eating and Physical Activity." *Annual Review of Public Health* 22 (2001): 309–335.

Friedman, B., S. P. Gordon, and J. B. Peers. "Effect of Neotraditional Neighborhood Design on Travel Characteristics." *Transportation Research Record* 1466 (1995): 63–70.

Friedman, M. S., K. E. Powell, L. Hutwagner, et al. "Impact of Changes in Transportation and Commuting Behaviors During the 1996 Summer Olympic Games in Atlanta on Air Quality and Childhood Asthma." *Journal of the American Medical Association* 285 (no. 7, 2001): 897–905.

Frumkin, H. "Urban Sprawl and Public Health." *Public Health Reports* 117 (2002): 201–217.

Gallo, A. E. "Food Advertising in the United States," in E. Frazao (ed.), *America's Eating Habits: Changes and Consequences.* Washington, DC: USDA/Economic Research Service, 1999.

Geller, A. L. "Smart Growth: A Prescription for Livable Cities." *American Journal of Public Health* 93 (2003): 1410–1415.

Giles-Corti, B., and R. J. Donovan. "The Relative Influence of Individual, Social and Physical Environment Determinants of Physical Activity." *Social Science and Medicine* 54 (2002): 1793–1812.

———. "Relative Influences of Individual, Social Environmental, and Physical Environmental Correlates of Walking." *American Journal of Public Health* 93 (2003): 1583–1589.

———. "Socioeconomic Status Differences in Recreational Physical Activity Levels and Real and Perceived Access to a Supportive Physical Environment." *Preventive Medicine* 35 (2002): 601–611.

Giles-Corti, B., S. Macintyre, J. P. Clarkson, et al. "Environmental and Lifestyle Factors Associated with Overweight and Obesity in Perth, Australia." *American Journal of Health Promotion* 18 (2003b): 93–102.

Gillham, O. *The Limitless City: A Primer on the Urban Sprawl Debate.* Washington, DC: Island Press, 2002.

Gorman, C. "Why So Many Are Getting Diabetes." *Time,* 8 December 2003.

Gorner, P. "Affluence Bringing Increase in Diabetes, Researcher Says." *Chicago Tribune,* 23 December 2003. www.defeatdiabetes.org/Articles/lifestyle030605.htm

Gortmaker, S. L., A. Must, A. M. Sobol, et al. "Television Viewing As a Cause of Increasing Obesity Among Children in the United States, 1986–1990." *Archives of Pediatric and Adolescent Medicine* 150 (1996): 356–362.

Greendale, G. A., E. Barrett-Connor, S. Edelstein, et al. "Lifetime Leisure Exercise and Osteoporosis: The Rancho Bernardo Study." *American Journal of Epidemiology* 141 (1995): 951–959.

Gregg, E. W., R. B. Gerzoff, C. J. Caspersen, et al. "Relationship of Walking to Mortality Among US Adults with Diabetes." *Archives of Internal Medicine* 163 (2003): 1440–1447.

Gustafson, D., E. Rothenberg, K. Blennow, et al. "An 18-Year Follow-up of Overweight and Risk of Alzheimer Disease." *Archives of Internal Medicine* 163 (2003): 1524–1528.

Hahn, R. A., S. M. Teutsch, R. B. Rothenberg, et al. "Excess Deaths from Nine Chronic Diseases in the United States, 1986." *Journal of the American Medical Association* 264 (1991): 2654–2659.

Harnik, P. "History of the Rail-Trail Movement." Rails-to-Trails Conservancy, 2005. www.railtrails.org/about/history.asp

Harrison, L., M. A. Brenna, and A. M. Levine. "Physical Activity Patterns and Body Mass Index Scores Among Military Service Members." *American Journal of Health Promotion* 15 (2000): 77–80.

Hart, S. I., and A. L. Spivak. *The Elephant in the Bedroom: Automobile Dependence and Denial, Impacts on the Economy and Environment.* Pasadena, CA: New Paradigm Books, 1993.

Heini, A. F., and R. L. Weinsier. "Divergent Trends in Obesity and Fat Intake Patterns: The American Paradox." *American Journal of Medicine* 102 (1997): 259–264.

Henry, J. "Too Fat to Get Fit: The Children Unable to Take Part in PE Class." News.Telegraph.co.uk, 16 March 2003. www.telegraph.co.uk/news/main.jhtml?xml=/news/2003/03/16/nfat16.xml

Hirschhorn, J. S. "Zoning Should Promote Public Health." *American Journal of Health Promotion* 18 (2004): 258–260.

Holland, AJA, R. W. Y. Liang, S. J. Singh, et al. "Driveway Motor Vehicle Injuries in Children." *Medical Journal of Australia* 173 (2000): 192–195.

Holtz Kay, J. *Asphalt Nation: How the Automobile Took Over America and How We Can Take It Back.* New York: Crown, 1997.

"Hospitals Feel New Costs of Obese Patients." Reuters, 18 December 2003. www.msnbc.com/Default.aspx?id=3751888&p1=0

Hu, F. B., G. A. Colditz, W. C. Willett, et al. "Television Watching and Other Sedentary Behaviors in Relation to Risk of Obesity and Type 2 Diabetes Mellitus in Women." *Journal of the American Medical Association* 289 (2003): 1785–1791.

Hu, F. B., M. F. Leitzmann, M. J. Stampfer, et al. "Physical Activity and Television Watching in Relation to Risk for Type 2 Diabetes Mellitus in Men." *Archives of Internal Medicine* 161 (2001): 1542–1548.

Hussain, R. "Hospitals Buy More Extra-Large Gear." *Chicago Sun-Times*, 13 January 2004.

Huttenmoser, M. "Children and Their Living Surroundings: Empirical Investigations into the Significance of Living Surroundings for the Everyday Life and Development of Children." *Children's Environments* 12 (1995): 403–413.

Illich, I. *Energy and Equity.* New York: HarperCollins, 1974.

Iwane, M., M. Arita, S. Tomimoto, et al. "Walking 10,000 Steps/Day or More Reduces Blood Pressure and Sympathetic Nerve Activity in Mild Essential Hypertension." *Hypertensive Research* 23 (2000): 573–580.

Jacobs, J. *The Death and Life of Great American Cities.* New York: Random House, 1961.

Jaffe, D. H., M. E. Singer, and A. A. Rimm. "Air Pollution and Emergency Department Visits for Asthma Among Ohio Medicaid Recipients, 1991–1996." *Environmental Research* 91 (2003): 21–28.

Jakicic, J. M., B. H. Marcus, K. I. Gallagher, et al. "Effect of Exercise Duration and Intensity on Weight Loss in Overweight, Sedentary Women." *Journal of the American Medical Association* 290 (2003): 1323–1330.

Janz, K. F., S. M. Levy, T. L. Burns, et al. "Fatness, Physical Activity, and Television Viewing in Children During the Adiposity Rebound Period: The Iowa Bone Development Study." *Preventive Medicine* 35 (2002): 563–571.

Jebb, S. A., and M. S. Moore. "Contribution of a Sedentary Lifestyle and Inactivity to the Etiology of Overweight and Obesity: Current Evidence and Research Issues." *Medicine and Science in Sports and Exercise* 31 (1999): S534–541.

Jedwab, J. "Getting to Work in North America's Major Cities and Dependence on Cars." Montreal, QC, Canada: Association for Canadian Studies, 2004. www.acs-aec.ca/Polls/locomotions.pdf

Joly, M. F., P. M. Foggin, and I. B. Pless. "Geographical and Socio-Ecological Variations of Traffic Accidents Among Children." *Social Science and Medicine* 33 (1991): 765–769.

Kahn, L. K., M. K. Serdula, B. A. Bowman, et al. "Use of Prescription Weight Loss Pills Among U.S. Adults in 1996–1998." *Annals of Internal Medicine* 134 (2001): 282–286.

Kaiser Family Foundation. "The Role of Media in Childhood Obesity." Menlo Park, CA: Kaiser Family Foundation, February 2004. www.kff.org/entmedia/entmedia022404pres.cfm

Kappelman T. *Marshall McLuhan: "The Medium Is the Message."* Richardson TX: Probe Ministries, 2001. www.leaderu.com/orgs/probe/docs/mcluhan.html

Katzmarzyk, P. T., N. Gledhill, and R. J. Shephard. "The Economic Burden of Physical Inactivity in Canada." *Canadian Medical Association Journal* 163 (2000): 1435–1440.

Kelley, G. A., K. S. Kelley, and Z. V. Tran. "Walking and Resting Blood Pressure in Adults: A Meta-Analysis." *Preventive Medicine* 33 (2001): 120–127.

Kennedy, M. F., and W. H. Meeuwisse. "Exercise Counselling by Family Physicians in Canada." *Preventive Medicine* 37 (2003): 226–232.

Kersh, R., and J. Morone. "The Politics of Obesity: Seven Steps to Government Action." *Health Affairs* 21 (2002): 142–153.

Kifer, K. "Is Cycling Dangerous?" Ken Kifer's Bike Pages, n.d. www.kenkifer.com/bikepages/health/risks.htm

Killingsworth, R. E. "Health Promoting Community Design: A New Paradigm to Promote Healthy and Active Communities." *American Journal of Health Promotion* 17 (2003): 169–170.

King, W. C., J. S. Brach, S. Belle, et al. "The Relationship Between Convenience of Destinations and Walking Levels in Older Women." *American Journal of Health Promotion* 18 (2003): 74–82.

Klesges, R. C., M. L. Shelton, and L. M. Klesges. "Effects of Television on Metabolic Rate: Potential Implications for Childhood Obesity." *Pediatrics* 91 (1993): 281–286.

Koepsell T., L. McCloskey, M. Wolf, et al. "Crosswalk Markings and the Risk of Pedestrian-Motor Vehicle Collisions in Older Pedestrians." *Journal of the American Medical Association* 288 (2002): 2136–2143.

Koplan, J. P., and W. H. Dietz. "Caloric Imbalance and Public Health Policy." *Journal of the American Medical Association* 282 (1999): 1579–1581.

Koslowsky, M., A. N. Kluger, and M. Reich. *Commuting Stress: Causes, Effects, and Methods of Coping.* New York: Plenum, 1995.

Kriel, R. L., M. E. Gormley, L. E. Krach, et al. "Automatic Garage Door Openers: Hazard for Children." *Pediatrics* 98 (1996): 770–773.

Kunstler, J. H. "Home from Nowhere." *Atlantic Monthly*, September 1996, 43–66. www.theatlantic.com/issues/96sep/kunstler.htm

———. *Home from Nowhere: Remaking Our Everyday World for the 21st Century.* Touchstone Books, 1998.

Kunzli, N., R. McConnell, D. Bates, et al. "Breathless in Los Angeles: The Exhausting Search for Clean Air." *American Journal of Public Health* 93 (2003): 1494–1499.

Laflamme, L., and F. Diderichsen. "Social differences in Traffic Injury Risks in Childhood and Youth: A Literature Review and Research Agenda." *Injury Prevention* 6 (2000): 293–298. ip.bmjjournals.com/cgi/content/full/6/4/293

Lakdawalla, D. N., J. Bhattacharya, and D. P. Goldman. "Are the Young Becoming More Disabled?" *Health Affairs* 23 (2004): 168–176.

Langlois, J. A., P. M. Keyl, J. M. Guralnik, et al. "Characteristics of Older Pedestrians Who Have Difficulty Crossing the Street." *American Journal of Public Health* 87 (1997): 393–397.

Laurin, D., R. Verreault, J. Lindsay, et al. "Physical Activity and Risk of Cognitive Impairment and Dementia in Elderly Persons." *Archives of Neurology* 58 (2001): 498–504.

Leden, L. "Pedestrian Risk Decrease with Pedestrian Flow: A Case Study Based on Data from Signalized Intersections in Hamilton, Ontario." *Accident Analysis and Prevention* 34 (2002): 457–464.

Lee, I., and R. S. Paffenbarger, Jr. "Associations of Light, Moderate, and Vigorous Intensity Physical Activity with Longevity." *American Journal of Epidemiology* 151 (2000): 293–299.

Lewis, D. E. "Overweight Workers Say They're Often Overlooked." *Boston Globe*, 21 September 2003. bostonworks.boston.com/globe/articles/092103_body.html

Leyden, K. M. "Social Capital and the Built Environment: The Importance of Walkable Neighborhoods." *American Journal of Public Health* 93 (2003): 1546–1551.

Lightstone, A. S., P. K. Dhillon, C. Peek-Asa, et al. "A Geographic Analysis of Motor Vehicle Collisions with Child Pedestrians in Long Beach, California: Comparing Intersection and Midblock Incident Locations." *Injury Prevention* 7 (2001): 155–160.

Litman, T. A. "Economic Value of Walkability." Victoria, BC, Canada: Victoria Transport Policy Institute, 2003. www.vtpi.org/walkability.pdf

———. "Evaluating Transportation Land Use Impacts." Victoria, BC, Canada: Victoria Transport Policy Institute, 2003. www.vtpi.org/landuse.pdf

———. "The Costs of Automobile Dependency and the Benefits of Balanced Transportation." Victoria, BC, Canada: Victoria Transport Policy Institute, 2002. www.landcentre.ca/lcframedoc.cfm?ID=4055 (PDF)

———. "Traffic Calming Benefits, Costs and Equity Impacts." Victoria Transport Policy Institute, Victoria, BC, Canada, 1999. www.vtpi.org/calming.pdf

Local Government Commission Center for Livable Communities. "The Economic Benefits of Walkable Communities." Sacramento, CA, 2004. www.lgc.org/freepub/land_use/factsheets/walk_to_money.html

Lofland, L. H. *The Public Realm: Exploring the City's Quintessential Social Territory.* New York: Aldine de Gruyter, 1998.

Lowry, R., H. Weschler, D. A. Galuska, et al. "Television Viewing and Its Associations with Overweight, Sedentary Lifestyle, and Insufficient Consumption of Fruits and Vegetables Among US High School Students: Differences by Race, Ethnicity, and Gender." *Journal of School Health* 72 (2002): 413–421.

Lucy W. H. "Mortality Risk Associated with Leaving Home: Recognizing the Relevance of the Built Environment." *American Journal of Public Health* 93 (2003): 1564–1569.

Ludwig, D. S., K. E. Peterson, and S. L. Gortmaker. "Relation Between Consumption of Sugar-Sweetened Drinks and Childhood Obesity: A Prospective, Observational Analysis." *Lancet* 357 (2001): 505–508.

Luepker, R. V. "How Physically Active Are American Children and What Can We Do About It?" *International Journal of Obesity* 23 (suppl. 2, 1999): S12–S17.

Macaluso, N. "Link Between Health and Sprawl Makes 'Smart' Growth Look Even Smarter." *Miami Herald,* 6 June 2003. Available at (registration required): www.miami.com/mld/miamiherald/59600236.htm

Macionis, J. J., and V. N. Parillo. *Cities and Urban Life,* 2nd ed. Upper Saddle River, NJ: Prentice Hall, 2000.

Madanipour, A. *Design of Urban Space: An Inquiry into a Socio-Spatial Process.* New York: Wiley, 1996.

Manson, J. E., P. J. Skerrett, P. Greenland, et al. "The Escalating Pandemics of Obesity and Sedentary Lifestyle: A Call to Action for Clinicians." *Archives of Internal Medicine* 164 (2004): 249–258.

Manson, J. E., P. Greenland, A. Z. LaCroix, et al. "Walking Compared with Vigorous Exercise for the Prevention of Cardiovascular Events in Women." *New England Journal of Medicine* 347 (2002): 716–724.

Martinez-Gonzalez, M. A., J. A. Martinez, F. B. Hu, et al. "Physical Inactivity, Sedentary Lifestyle and Obesity in the European Union." *International Journal of Obesity* 23 (1999): 1192–1201.

McCann, B., and B. DeLille. "Mean Streets 2000: Pedestrian Safety, Health and Federal Transportation Spending, a Transportation and Quality of Life Campaign Report." Washington, DC: Surface Transportation Policy Project, 2000. www.transact.org/report.asp?id=132

McCann, B., and R. Ewing. "Measuring the Health Effects of Sprawl: A National Analysis of Physical Activity, Obesity and Chronic Disease." Washington, DC: Smart Growth America, Surface Transportation Policy Project, 2003. www.transact.org/report.asp?id=229

McLuhan, M. *Understanding Media: The Extensions of Man.* New York: McGraw-Hill, 1964.

McTiernan, A., C. Kooperberg, E. White, et al. "Recreational Physical Activity and the Risk of Breast Cancer in Postmenopausal Women." *Journal of the American Medical Association* 290 (2003): 1331–1336.

Merom, D., A. Bauman, P. Vita, et al. "An Environmental Intervention to Promote Walking and Cycling: The Impact of a Newly Constructed Rail Trail in Western Sydney." *Preventive Medicine* 36 (2003): 235–242.

Mid-Atlantic Integrated Assessment (MAIA). "Urban Sprawl." Washington, DC: U.S. Environmental Protection Agency, 2004. www.epa.gov/maia/html/sprawl.html

Mindell, J., L. Sheridan, M. Joffe, et al. "Health Impact Assessment As an Agent of Policy Change: Improving the Health Impacts of the Mayor of London's Draft Transport Strategy." *Journal of Epidemiology and Community Health* 58 (2004): 169–174.

Mokdad, A. H., J. S. Marks, D. F. Stroup, et al. "Actual Causes of Death in the United States, 2000." *Journal of the American Medical Association* 291 (2004): 1238–1245.

Mokdad, A. H., B. A. Bowman, E. S. Ford, et al. "The Continuing Epidemics of Obesity and Diabetes in the United States." *Journal of the American Medical Association* 286 (2001): 1195–1200.

Mokdad, A. H., M. K. Serdula, W. H. Dietz, et al. "The Spread of the Obesity Epidemic in the United States, 1991–1998." *Journal of the American Medical Association* 282 (1999): 1519–1522.

Moore, M. T. "City, Suburban Designs Could Be Bad for Your Health." *USA Today,* 22 April 2003. usatoday.com/news/health/2003-04-22-walk-cover_x.htm

Moreau, K. L., R. Degarmo, J. Langley, et al. "Increasing Daily Walking Lowers Blood Pressure in Postmenopausal Women." *Medicine and Science in Sports and Exercise* 33 (2001): 1825–1831.

Morris, J. N., and A. E. Hardman. "Walking to Health." *Sports Medicine* 23 (1997): 306–332.

Mueller, B.A., F. P. Rivara, S. M. Lii, et al. "Environmental Factors and the Risk for Childhood Pedestrian-Motor Vehicle Collision Occurrence." *American Journal of Epidemiology* 132 (1990): 550–560.

Mumford, L. *The City in History: Its Origins, Its Transformations, and Its Prospects.* New York: Harcourt, Brace and World, 1961.

Must, A., J. Spadano, E. H. Coakly, et al. "The Disease Burden Associated with Overweight and Obesity." *Journal of the American Medical Association* 282 (1999): 1523–1529.

Nadler, E.P., A. P. Courcoulas, M. J. Gardner, et al. "Driveway Injuries in Children: Risk Factors, Morbidity, and Mortality." *Pediatrics* 108 (2001): 326–328.

Narayan, K. M., J. P. Boyle, T. J. Thompson, et al. "Lifetime Risk for Diabetes Mellitus in the United States." *Journal of the American Medical Association* 290 (no. 14, 2003): 1884–1890.

Nash, J. M. "Obesity Goes Global." *Time,* 25 August 2003. www.time.com/time/archive/preview/from_search/ 0,10987,1101030825-476417,00.html

National Diabetes Information Clearinghouse, "National Diabetes Statistics." diabetes.niddk.nih.gov/dm/pubs/statistics/#14

Nestle, M., and M. F. Jacobson. "Halting the Obesity Epidemic: A Public Health Approach." *Public Health Reports* 115 (2000): 12–24.

Nolte, R., S. C. Franckowiak, C. J. Crespo, et al. "U.S. Military Weight Standards: What Percentage of U.S. Young Adults Meet the Current Standards?" *American Journal of Medicine* 113 (2002): 486–490.

Norris, G., S. N. YoungPong, J. Q. Koenig, et al. "An Association Between Fine

Particles and Asthma Emergency Department Visits for Children in Seattle." *Environmental Health Perspectives* 107 (1999): 489–493.

"Obesity Factfile," *Primary Care—NHS Magazine*, June 2002. www.nhs.uk/nhsmagazine/primarycare/archives/jun2002/feature2b.asp

"The Obesity Industry: Big Business." *Economist*, 27 September 2003.

O'Connor, A. "Now You and Your Canine Companion Can Both Shed— Pounds, That Is." *National Post*, 23 November 2004.

Ogden, C. L., K. M. Flegal, M. D. Carroll, et al. "Prevalence and Trends in Overweight Among U.S. Children and Adolescents, 1999–2000." *Journal of the American Medical Association* 288 (2002): 1728–1732.

Owen, N., N. Humpel, E. Leslie, et al. "Understanding Environmental Influences on Walking: Review and Research Agenda." *American Journal of Preventive Medicine* 27 (2004): 67–76.

Paluska, S. A., and T. L. Schwenk. "Physical Activity and Mental Health: Current Concepts." *Sports Medicine* 29 (2000): 167–180.

Paris, R. M., S. A. Bedno, M. R. Krauss, et al. "Weighing in on Type 2 Diabetes in the Military: Characteristics of U.S. Military Personnel at Entry Who Develop Type 2 Diabetes." *Diabetes Care* 24 (2001): 1894–1898.

Pate, R. R., M. Pratt, S. N. Blair, et al. "Physical Activity and Public Health: A Recommendation from the Centers for Disease Control and Prevention and the American College of Sports Medicine." *Journal of the American Medical Association* 273 (1995): 402–407.

Pate, R. R., G. W. Heath, M. Dowda, et al. "Associations Between Physical Activity and Other Health Behaviors in a Representative Sample of US Adolescents." *American Journal of Public Health* 86 (1996): 1577–1581.

Paulos, E., and E. Goodman. "Familiar Stranger Project: Anxiety, Comfort, and Play in Public Places." Berkeley, CA: Intel Research Laboratory at Berkeley, 2004. berkeley.intel-research.net/paulos/research/familiarstranger

Pedestrian and Bicycle Information Center. "Growing Demand for Safe Walking and Bicycling: A Four Year Report." Chapel Hill, NC, January 2003.

Peeters, A., J. J. Barendregt, F. Willekens, et al. "Obesity in Adulthood and Its Consequences for Life Expectancy: A Life-Table Analysis." *Annals of Internal Medicine* 138 (no. 1, 2003): 24–32.

Phillips, E. B. *City Lights: Urban–Suburban Life in the Global Society*, 2nd ed. New York: Oxford University Press, 1996.

Pollard, K. "Going to Work: Americans' Commuting Patterns in 2000." Population Reference Bureau, 2004. www.prb.org/AmeristatTemplate.cfm?Section=2000Census1&template=/ ContentManagement/ContentDisplay.cfm&ContentID=7839

Pollard, T. "Policy Prescriptions for Healthier Communities." *American Journal of Health Promotion* 18 (2003): 109–113.

Poston, W. S., and J. P. Foreyt. "Obesity Is an Environmental Issue." *Atherosclerosis* 146 (1999): 201–209.

Powell, K. E., and S. N. Blair. "The Public Health Burdens of Sedentary Living Habits: Theoretical but Realistic Estimates." *Medicine and Science in Sports and Exercise* 26 (1994): 851–856.

Pratt, M., C. A. Macera, and C. Blanton. "Levels of Physical Activity and Inactivity in Children and Adults in the United States: Current Evidence and Research Issues." *Medicine and Science in Sports and Exercise* 31 (1999): S526–S533.

Prentice, A. M., and S. A. Jebb. "Obesity in Britain: Gluttony or Sloth?" *British Medical Journal* 311 (1995): 437–439. www.ncbi.nlm.nih.gov/entrez/query.fcgi?cmd=Retrieve&db=PubMed& list_uids=7640595&dopt=Abstract

Pucher, J. "Renaissance of Public Transport in the United States?" *Transportation Quarterly* 56 (2002): 33–49.

———. "Transportation Paradise: Realm of the Nearly Perfect Automobile?" *Transportation Quarterly* 53 (1999):115–120.

Pucher, J., and L. Dijkstra. "Promoting Safe Walking and Cycling to Improve Public Health: Lessons from the Netherlands and Germany." *American Journal of Public Health* 93 (2003): 1509–1516.

Pucher, J., C. Komanoff, and P. Schimek. "Bicycling Renaissance in North America? Recent Trends and Alternative Policies to Promote Bicycling." *Transportation Research* 33 (nos. 7/8, 1999): 625–654. www.vtpi.org/pucher3.pdf

Putnam, R. D. *Bowling Alone: The Collapse and Revival of American Community.* New York: Simon and Schuster, 2000.

Rafferty, A. P., M. J. Reeves, H. B. McGee, et al. "Physical Activity Patterns Among Walkers and Compliance with Public Health Recommendations." *Medicine and Science in Sports and Exercise* 34 (2002): 1255–1261.

Reichholf, J. H. *L'émergence de l'homme.* Paris: Champs Flammarion, 1990.

"Researcher Links Obesity, Food Portions." Yahoo! News, 3 January 2004. www.skinnykat.com/litter/archives/2004/01/researcher_link.html

Retting, R. A., S. A. Ferguson, and A. T. McCartt. "A Review of Evidence-Based Traffic Engineering Measures Designed to Reduce Pedestrian–Motor Vehicle Crashes." *American Journal of Public Health* 93 (2003): 1456–1463.

Retting, R. A., B. N. Persaud, P. E. Garder, et al. "Crash and Injury Reduction Following Installation of Roundabouts in the United States." *American Journal of Public Health* 2001: 91: 628–631.

Revill, J. "A Deadly Slice of American Pie." *The Guardian,* 20 September 2003. observer.guardian.co.uk/focus/story/0,6903,1046514,00.html

Robbins, A. S., S. Y. Chao, C. R. Russ, et al. "Costs of Excess Body Weight

Among Active Duty Personnel, U.S. Air Force, 1997." *Military Medicine* 167 (2002): 393–397.

Roberts, I. "International Trends in Pedestrian Injury Mortality." *Archives of Diseases in Children* 68 (1993a): 190–192.

———. "What Does a Decline in Child Pedestrian Injury Rates Mean?" *American Journal of Public Health* 85 (1995): 268.

———. "Why Have Child Pedestrian Death Rates Fallen?" *British Medical Journal* 306 (1993b): 1737–1739.

Roberts, I., J. Carlin, C. Bennett, et al. "An International Study of the Exposure of Children to Traffic." *Injury Prevention* 3 (1997): 89–93.

Roberts, I., and C. Coggan. "Blaming Children for Child Pedestrian Injuries." *Social Science and Medicine* 38 (1994): 749–753.

Roberts, I., and I. Crombie. "Child Pedestrian Deaths: Sensitivity to Traffic Volume, Evidence from the USA." *Journal of Epidemiology and Community Health* 49 (1995): 186–188.

Roberts, I., R. Marshall, and T. Lee-Joe. "The Urban Traffic Environment and the Risk of Child Pedestrian Injury: A Case-Crossover Approach." *Epidemiology* 6 (1995): 169–171.

Roberts, I., R. Norton, and R. Jackson. "Driveway-related Child Pedestrian Injuries: A Case-Control Study." *Pediatrics* 95 (1995): 405–408.

Roberts, I., R. Norton, R. Jackson, et al. "Effect of Environmental Factors on Risk of Injury of Child Pedestrians by Motor Vehicles: A Case-Control Study." *British Medical Journal* 310 (1995): 91–94.

Roberts, I., H. Owen, P. Lumb, et al. "Pedalling Health: Health Benefits of a Modal Transport Shift." Birmingham, England: Birmingham University Bicycle User Group, 1996. www.cycling.bham.ac.uk/pdf/cyhealth.pdf

Robinson, D. L. "Head Injuries and Bicycle Helmet Laws." *Accident Analysis and Prevention* 28 (1996): 463–475.

Robinson, G. "Overweight America" (letter). *Consumer Reports,* March 2004, 10.

Robinson, T. N. "Television Viewing and Childhood Obesity." *Pediatric Clinics of North America* 48 (2001): 1017–1025.

Rooney, B., K. Smalley, J. Larson, et al. "Is Knowing Enough? Increasing Physical Activity by Wearing a Pedometer." *Wisconsin Medical Journal* 102 (2003): 31–36.

Rudovsky, B. *Streets for People: A Primer for Americans.* New York: Doubleday, 1969.

Salmon, J., A. Bauman, D. Crawford, et al. "The Association Between Television Viewing and Overweight Among Australian Adults Participating in Varying Levels of Leisure-Time Physical Activity." *International Journal of Obesity and Related Metabolic Disorders* 24 (2000): 600–606.

Sampson, R. J., S. W. Raudenbush, and F. Earls. "Neighborhoods and Violent Crime: A Multi-Level Study of Collective Efficacy." *Science* 277 (1997): 918–924.

Sanmartin, C., E. Ng, D. Blackwell, et al. "Joint Canada/United States Survey of Health, 2002–03." Statistics Canada, Catalogue no. 82M0022-XIE, Ottawa, June 2004. www.cdc.gov/nchs/about/major/nhis/jcush_mainpage.htm

Schmidt, C. W. "Obesity: A Weighty Issue for Children." *Environmental Health Perspectives* 111 (2003): A701–A707.

Schwimmer, J. B., T. M. Burwinkle, and J. W. Varni. Health-related Quality of Life of Severely Obese Children and Adolescents. *Journal of the American Medical Association* 289 (2003): 1813–1819.

Sealy, G. "Beyond Baby Fat: As Childhood Obesity Grows, Experts Say the Stakes Can't Be Higher." ABCNews.com, 30 September 2003. www24.homepage.villanova.edu/elias.nure/f4k/articles/ Beyond_Baby_Fat.pdf

———. "Just Do It: Many Schools Cutting Gym Class." ABCNews.com, 30 September 2003. www.ihpra.org/ABCNEWS_com%20%20No%20Sweat%20When% 20Gym%20Class%20Cut.htm

Seidell, J. C. "Societal and Personal Costs of Obesity." *Experimental and Clinical Endocrinology in Diabetes* 106 (1998): 7–9.

Sierra Club. "Sprawl: the Dark Side of the American Dream." Sierra Club, 1998. www.sierraclub.org/sprawl/report98/report.asp

———. "Smart Choices or Sprawling Growth: A 50-State Survey of Development." Sierra Club, 2000. www.sierraclub.org/sprawl

Singer, D. G. "A Time to Re-Examine the Role of Television in Our Lives." *American Psychologist* 38 (1983): 815–816.

Slentz, C. A., B. D. Duscha, J. L. Johnson, et al. "Effects of the Amount of Exercise on Body Weight, Body Composition, and Measures of Central Obesity." *Archives of Internal Medicine* 164 (2004): 31–39.

Solnit, R. *Wanderlust: A History of Walking.* New York: Penguin, 2000.

Sparling, P. B., E. Owen, E. V. Lambert, et al. "Promoting Physical Activity: The New Imperative for Public Health." *Health Education Research* 15 (2000): 367–376.

Staples, B. "How the Most Dangerous Pedestrian in Los Angeles Got a Makeover." *New York Times* 26 July 2003. Available for purchase at: www.nytimes.com/2003/07/26/opinion/26SAT4.html?ex=1060274880&ei= 1&en=...

Staunton, C. E., D. Hubsmith, and W. Kallins. "Promoting Safe Walking and Biking to School: The Marin County Success Story." *American Journal of Public Health* 93 (2003): 1431–1434.

Stevenson, M. R., K. D. Jamrozik, and J. Spittle. "A Case-Control Study of Traffic Risk Factors and Child Pedestrian Injury." *International Journal of Epidemiology* 24 (1995): 957–964.

"Study Shows Massive Tree Loss in U.S. Cities." Reuters, ENN News, 18 September 2003. www.ufei.org/news.lasso

Sturm, R. "The Effects of Obesity, Smoking, and Drinking on Medical Problems and Costs." *Health Affairs* 21 (2002): 245–253.

———. "Increases in Clinically Severe Obesity in the United States, 1986–2000." *Archives of Internal Medicine* 163 (2003): 2146–2148.

Surface Transportation Policy Project. "Aggressive Driving: Where You Live Matters." Washington, DC: Surface Transportation Policy Project, January 1999. www.transact.org/report.asp?id=56

———. "Americans' Attitudes Toward Walking and Creating Better Walking Communities." Washington, DC: Surface Transportation Policy Project, April 2003. www.transact.org/report.asp?id=205

———. "Changing Direction." Washington, DC: Surface Transportation Policy Project, January 2000. www.transact.org/report.asp?id=163

———. "High Mileage Moms: The Report." Washington, DC: Surface Transportation Policy Project, 2002. www.transact.org/report.asp?id=182

———. "Transportation and Biodiversity." Washington, DC: Surface Transportation Policy Project, 2003. www.transact.org/library/factsheets/biodiversity.asp

———. "Transportation and Economic Prosperity." Washington, DC: Surface Transportation Policy Project, 2003. www.transact.org/library/factsheets/prosperity.asp

———. "Transportation and the Environment." Washington, DC: Surface Transportation Policy Project, 2003. www.transact.org/library/factsheets/environment.asp

———. "Transportation and Health." Washington, DC: Surface Transportation Policy Project, 2003. www.transact.org/library/factsheets/health.asp

———. "Transportation Costs and the American Dream." Washington, DC: Surface Transportation Policy Project, July 2003. www.transact.org/report.asp?id=224

———. "Transportation Data from the 2000 Census." Washington, DC: Surface Transportation Policy Project, 2002. www.transact.org/report.asp?id=188

———. "The 2002 Summary of Safe Routes to School Programs in the United States." Washington, DC: Surface Transportation Policy Project, 2002. www.transact.org/report.asp?id=49

———. "Why Are the Roads So Congested?" Washington, DC: Surface Transportation Policy Project, 1999. www.transact.org/report.asp?id=63

Surface Transportation Policy Project California. "The Link Between Traffic Congestion and Sprawl." Surface Transportation Policy Project California, n.d. www.transact.org/Ca/congestion6.htm

Swinburn, B., G. Egger, and F. Raza. "Dissecting Obesogenic Environments: The Development and Application of a Framework for Identifying and Prioritizing Environmental Interventions for Obesity." *Preventive Medicine* 29 (1999): 563–570.

Takano, T, K. Nakamura, and M. Watanabe. "Urban Residential Environments and Senior Citizens' Longevity in Megacity Areas: The Importance of Walkable Green Spaces." *Journal of Epidemiology and Community Health* 56 (2002): 913–918.

Tanner, L. "Study: We're Eating Ourselves to Death." *My Way News*, 2004. apnews.myway.com/article/20040309/D8173CP00.html

Texas Transportation Institute. "2003 Urban Mobility Study." Available at: mobility.tamu.edu/ums/report

Thompson, Don. "Pets Mirror Nation's Obesity Problem, Data Shows." *San Mateo County Times*, 22 December 2003.

Thompson, David., J. Edelsberg, K. L. Kinsey, et al. "Estimated Economic Costs of Obesity to U.S. Business." *American Journal of Health Promotion* 13 (1998): 120–127.

Tolbert, P. E., J. A. Mulholland, D. L. MacIntosh, et al. "Air Quality and Paediatric Emergency Room Visits for Asthma in Atlanta, Georgia, USA." *American Journal of Epidemiology* 151 (2000): 798–810.

Townsend, M., and D. Campbell. "Britain's Battle of the Bulge." *Observer*, 21 September 2003. observer.guardian.co.uk/focus/story/0,6903,1046510,00.html

Transportation Research Board. "The Relative Risks of School Travel: A National Perspective and Guidance for Local Community Risk Assessment." Special Report 269. Washington, DC: Transportation Research Board, 2002. www.trb.org/news/blurb_detail.asp?id=673

Tremblay, M. S., and J. D. Willms. "Secular Trends in the Body Mass Index of Canadian Children." *Canadian Medical Association Journal* 163 (2001): 1429–1433.

Trudeau, F., L. Laurencelle, J. Tremblay, et al. "Daily Primary School Physical Education: Effects on Physical Activity During Adult Life." *Medicine and Science in Sports and Exercise* 31 (1999): 111–117.

Tucker, L. A., and M. Bagwell. "Television Viewing and Obesity in Adult Females." *American Journal of Public Health* 81 (1991): 908–911.

Tucker, L. A., and G. M. Friedman. "Television Viewing and Obesity in Adult Males." *American Journal of Public Health* 79 (1989): 516–518.

Tyre, P. "Getting Rid of Extra Pounds." *Newsweek*, 8 December 2003. surgerynews.net/news/1203/weight12301.htm

U.S. Department of Health and Human Services. "Physical Activity and Health: A Report of the Surgeon General." Atlanta, GA: U.S. Department of Health and Human Services, Centers for Disease Control and Prevention,

National Center for Chronic Disease Prevention and Health Promotion, 1996. www.cdc.gov/nccdphp/sgr/sgr.htm

U.S. Department of Transportation. "National Bicycling and Walking Study, Case Study No 1: Reasons Why Bicycling and Walking Are and Are Not Being Used More Extensively As Travel Modes." Washington, DC: Federal Highway Administration, 1992. Publication No. FHWA-PD-92-041. www.bikewalk.org/assets/pdf/CASE.PDF

"US Kids Show Early Signs of Heart Disease." NewScientist.com, 10 November 2003. www.newscientist.com/article.ns?id=dn4364&print=true

Van Vliet, P., M. Knape, J. de Hartog, et al. "Motor Vehicle Exhaust and Chronic Respiratory Symptoms in Children Living Near Freeways." *Environmental Research* 74 (1997): 122–132.

Vellinga, M. L. "Dream Homes or Rural Nightmares?" *Sacramento Bee*, 25 January 2004. www.sactaqc.org/Resources/Literature/LandUse/Ranchettes_Wilton.htm

"Vending Machine Controversy: Is the Student Body Buying Too Many Snacks?" ABCNews.com, 28 October 2003. www.fan4kids.com/articles/Vending_Machine_Controversy.pdf

Victoria Transport Policy Institute. *Transportation Demand Management Encyclopedia*. Victoria, BC, Canada, Victoria Transport Policy Institute, 2003. Online TDM Encyclopedia available at www.vtpi.org/tdm/tdm20.htm

Visscher, T. L. S., and J. Seidell. "The Public Health Impact of Obesity." *Annual Review of Public Health* 22 (2001): 355–375.

Vita, A. J., R. B. Terry, H. B. Hubert, et al. "Aging, Health Risks, and Cumulative Disability." *New England Journal of Medicine* 338 (1998): 1035–1041.

Wang, G., Z. J. Zheng, G. Heath, et al. "Economic Burden of Cardiovascular Disease Associated with Excess Body Weight in U.S. Adults." *American Journal of Preventive Medicine* 23 (2002): 1–6.

Wardlaw, M. J. "Three Lessons for a Better Cycling Future." *British Medical Journal* 321 (2000): 1582–1585. bmj.com/cgi/content/full/321/7276/1582

Wazana, A., V. L. Rynard, P. Raina, et al. "Are Child Pedestrians at Increased Risk of Injury on One-Way Compared to Two-Way Streets?" *Canadian Journal of Public Health* 91 (2000): 201–206.

Weiland, S. K., K. A. Mundt, A. Ruckmann, et al. "Self-Reported Wheezing and Allergic Rhinitis in Children and Traffic Density on Street of Residence." *Annals of Epidemiology* 4 (1994): 243–247.

Weinhold, B. "Don't Breathe and Drive?" *Environmental Health Perspectives* 109 (no. 9, 2001): A422–A427.

Weuve, J., J. H. Kang, J. E. Manson, et al. "Physical Activity, Including Walking, and Cognitive Function in Older Women." *Journal of the American Medical Association* 292 (2004): 1454–1461.

Wheatly, M. "How IT Fixed London's Traffic Woes." *CIO Magazine*, 15 July 2003. www.cio.com/archive/071503/london.html

Wilhelm, M., and B. Ritz. "Residential Proximity to Traffic and Adverse Birth Outcomes in Los Angeles County, California, 1994–1996." *Environmental Health Perspectives* 111 (2003): 207–216.

Wilkinson, B., and P. Jacobsen. "Why Transportation Is a Health Issue." National Center for Bicycling and Walking, August 2002. www.bikewalk.org/assets/pdf/Why_Transportation_is_a_Health_Issue_pdf

Williams-Derry, C. "Who Is the Smart Growth Leader? Hint: It's Not Portland." Michigan Land Use Institute, Elm Street Writers Group, 12 March 2002. www.mlui.org/growthmanagement/fullarticle.asp?fileid=16377

Winn, D.G., P. F. Agran, and D. N. Castillo. "Pedestrian Injuries to Children Younger Than 5 Years of Age." *Pediatrics* 88 (1991): 776–782.

Wjst, M., P. Reitmeir, S. Dold, et al. "Road Traffic and Adverse Effects on Respiratory Health in Children." *British Medical Journal* 307 (1993): 596–600.

Wolf, A. M., and G. A. Colditz. "Current Estimates of the Economic Cost of Obesity in the United States." *Obesity Research* 6 (1998): 97–106.

Wong, S. L., P. T. Katzmarzyk, N. Z. Nichaman, et al. "Cardiorespiratory Fitness Is Associated with Lower Abdominal Fat Independent of Body Mass Index." *Medicine and Science in Sports and Exercise* 36 (2004): 286–291.

Zegeer, C. V., C. Seiderman, P. Lagerwey, et al. "Pedestrian Facilities Users Guide: Providing Safety and Mobility." McLean, VA: U.S. Department of Transportation, Federal Highway Administration, 2002. Publication No. FHWA-RD-01-102.

INDEX

Check Out These Other Vital Health Titles!

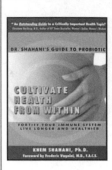
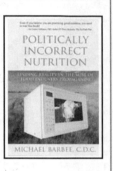
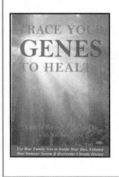